KU-753-097

the**facts**

Motor neuron disease

KEVIN TALBOT

Clinical Senior Lecturer, Department of Clinical Neurology,
University of Oxford, and Director, MND Care Centre,
John Radcliffe Hospital, Oxford, UK

RACHAEL MARSDEN

Motor Neuron Disease Specialist Nurse, Oxford Centre for
Enablement, and Coordinator of the Oxford Motor Neuron
Disease Care Centre, Oxford, UK

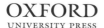

OXFORD
UNIVERSITY PRESS

OXFORD
UNIVERSITY PRESS

Great Clarendon Street, Oxford OX2 6DP

Oxford University Press is a department of the University of Oxford.
It furthers the University's objective of excellence in research, scholarship,
and education by publishing worldwide in

Oxford New York

Auckland Cape Town Dar es Salaam Hong Kong Karachi
Kuala Lumpur Madrid Melbourne Mexico City Nairobi
New Delhi Shanghai Taipei Toronto

With offices in

Argentina Austria Brazil Chile Czech Republic France Greece
Guatemala Hungary Italy Japan South Korea Poland Portugal
Singapore Switzerland Thailand Turkey Ukraine Vietnam

Oxford is a registered trade mark of Oxford University Press
in the UK and in certain other countries

Published in the United States
by Oxford University Press Inc., New York

British Library Cataloguing in Publication Data

Data available

Library of Congress Cataloging in Publication Data

Data available

Typeset by Newgen Imaging Systems (P) Ltd., Chennai, India
Printed in China
on acid-free paper by
Phoenix Offset

ISBN 978–0–19–920691–9 (Pbk.: alk paper)

10 9 8 7 6 5 4 3 2 1

Whilst every effort has been made to ensure that the contents of this book are as complete,
accurate and-up-to-date as possible at the date of writing, Oxford University Press is not able
to give any guarantee or assurance that such is the case. Readers are urged to take appropriately
qualified medical advice in all cases. The information in this book is intended to be useful to
the general reader, but should not be used as a means of self-diagnosis or for the prescription of
medication.

the**facts**

Motor neuron disease

Contents

Contents

Preface

Why did we write this book?

We decided to write this book because our daily experience of caring for patients with motor neuron disease (MND) is dominated by the exchange of information. Access to specialist care for people living with MND is becoming increasingly available, and the work of the Motor Neuron Disease Association in the UK and equivalent organizations elsewhere is transforming support for patients and carers. Information on the Internet, though it comes with a 'health warning', is readily accessible and can be very valuable. However, we feel that a book drawing on the detailed experience from a clinic dedicated to the diagnosis and management of MND would be of value to people living with MND.

Who is this book for?

This book is primarily for our patients and for their friends, relatives, and carers. However, the level of understanding of the disease among patients is often very sophisticated, and we have therefore written this book to a level of detail that we hope makes it useful to allied health professionals, especially the majority that only see a few MND patients in their working lives.

How to use this book?

Living with MND is a journey with many ups and downs. Most people want specific information which relates to their needs at a particular time but do not wish to be bombarded with information which seems more relevant to a later stage and may even appear threatening. One of the most difficult tasks in writing this book has been to devise a structure which fits with the different stages of the disease. We have tried to order the chapters so that they can be read in isolation and so that the early chapters reflect the concerns and questions which we hear from patients early in their disease. We suggest that patients who are newly diagnosed with MND will find Chapters 1–3 helpful as an initial source of information.

Kevin Talbot
Rachael Marsden

1

What is motor neuron disease?

Motor neurons are specialized nerve cells in the brain and spinal cord which transmit the electrical signals to muscles for the generation of movement. Two sorts of cells are required and, although it is an oversimplification, one can think of these as being like two switches in an electrical circuit (Fig. 1.1). The **upper motor neuron** starts at the top of the brain in an area called the motor cortex and travels down to the spinal cord to connect at different levels with the cells known as **lower motor neurons**. These cells in turn travel out of the spinal cord (e.g. along our arms and legs) and connect to muscle. If motor neurons are damaged or die, the main consequence is difficulty with voluntary movement.

In **motor neuron disease (MND)**, also known as **amyotrophic lateral sclerosis (ALS)**, motor neurons undergo progressive degeneration and die. The consequences for motor function differ depending on the extent to which upper and lower motor neurons are affected by degeneration. Figure 1.1 shows that lower motor neurons send out a long process, called the axon, to muscle. If this contact between the nerve and muscle is broken (e.g. if the nerve is cut or if the motor neuron dies), the muscle becomes thinner (a process known as muscle wasting or **atrophy**), the muscle loses its normal tone (i.e. becomes floppy) and weakness is inevitable. Although the main function of upper motor neurons is to initiate movement, much of the downward 'traffic' from the brain provides a moderating influence or 'brake' on muscle contraction. Therefore, if these upper motor neurons degenerate, the consequence is that limbs become stiffer (this is known as **spasticity**). The loss of function in MND/ALS is due to a mixture of weakness and stiffness of muscle.

Who is affected by MND/ALS?

Motor neuron degeneration affects 1 in 50 000 people in the population at large. This means that for every 100 000 people in the UK, two people will develop MND per year. At the individual level, approximately 1 in 1000 death certificates records MND as the cause of death. This can be put in perspective

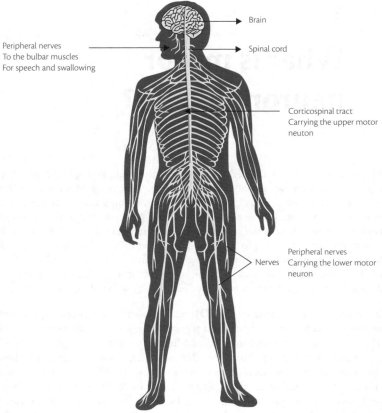

Brain

Peripheral nerves
To the bulbar muscles
For speech and swallowing

Spinal cord

Corticospinal tract
Carrying the upper motor
neuton

Nerves

Peripheral nerves
Carrying the lower motor
neuron

Figure 1.1 The anatomical pathways controlling movement. Voluntary movement is controlled by pathways which arise in upper motor neurons at the top of the brain. These travel to the spinal cord and connect with lower motor neurons which connect directly to muscle to activate movement.

by comparing stroke (which will affect 1 in 3 of all people at some time in their life) and all forms of cancer (the cause of death 1 in 4 people). In most cases, the reason that particular individuals get MND is a mystery. One thing that is clear is that the chance of MND developing increases with age. The average age at which people develop the disease is between 60 and 65 years of age, and it becomes more likely as people age further. Although currently a relatively rare disease compared with cancer, heart attacks or stroke, it will become more prevalent as the population ages. Currently there are about 5000–6000 people with MND in the UK at any one time and about 25 000–30 000 in the USA. The proportion of the population over the age of 65 is set at least to double over the next 50 years, with obvious consequences for the number of people with MND. The association of MND/ALS with ageing is similar to that of other age-related neurodegenerative diseases such as dementia or Parkinson's disease. This is not meant to imply that they have the same cause but simply that each of these diseases may have in common a failure of particular parts of the nervous system to adapt to the ageing process. This is one component of the cause of neurodegeneration, but clearly not the whole story.

Another striking feature of this disease is that men are affected about one and a half times more commonly than women. This is a consistent finding across specialist MND clinics throughout the world, and is therefore likely to be a meaningful clue to what makes particular people susceptible. For example, it has been proposed that there are differences in the way that motor neurons respond to hormones such as oestrogen.

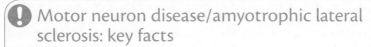 Motor neuron disease/amyotrophic lateral sclerosis: key facts

- MND is one of a group of age-related neurodegenerative diseases

- The population incidence is 1 in 50 000 and the individual lifetime risk is 1 in 400

- The number of people with MND/ALS in the UK = 7000, USA = 30 000

- Men are affected one and half times as often as women

- The average age of onset is about 60 years

- In 10 per cent of patients there is a family history, indicating that the disease is being caused by a variant of a gene which is passed through the generations

- The first symptoms arise either in the limbs (spinal onset) or in the muscles of speech and swallowing (bulbar onset)

- There are no specific tests to make a diagnosis of MND, which depends on the opinion of an expert neurologist

What are the first symptoms?

Approximately 70 per cent of patients with MND present with symptoms in the limbs. This is usually referred to as **spinal onset** MND on the assumption that the disease begins in the spinal cord, though this is probably an oversimplification. Most of the remaining patients present with difficulty with speech and/or swallowing, which is referred to as **bulbar onset** disease. The 'bulb' that is referred to here is another name for the brainstem (Fig. 1.1), the part of the central nervous system which is at the junction of the brain and spinal cord and contains the cell bodies of the lower motor neurons supplying the muscles of the palate, tongue, mouth and face.

Neurologists use various aspects of the physical examination to distinguish upper motor neuron from lower motor neuron damage, and to decide which regions of the body are affected. When lower motor neurons are damaged, the connecting muscle is wasted and weak. The wasting is often, but not always, accompanied by chaotic flickering of muscle called **fasciculation**, which is interpreted as a sign that muscle has lost its nervous connection. Doctors place a lot of emphasis on fasciculation in diagnosing MND, but as we shall see below it can occur in other situations. An example of a common pattern of symptoms with spinal onset ALS is wasting and weakness of the hand leading to difficulty in fine coordination (e.g. doing up buttons) and in hand grip (e.g. frequent dropping of objects). Alternatively, if the lower limb is affected, patients will complain that their foot 'drops', leading to tripping. When upper motor neurons are damaged, the affected muscle groups become stiff because the brain cannot provide the inhibition necessary for normal limb control, resulting in difficulty in coordinating walking and in responding to sudden changes in movement. People with stiff legs therefore often feel unstable, trip and have generally impaired mobility. In the arms, stiffness leads to slowness and clumsiness with fine movements such as picking up small objects. MND affecting the limbs, whatever the combination of upper or lower motor neuron damage, usually affects one side of the body more than the other early in the disease. The muscles of speech and swallowing (which are many and complex) can be affected by lower motor neuron damage, in which case the tongue is wasted and weak and speech sounds 'flabby'. In isolation this is relatively rare and, more commonly there is a mixture of lower motor neuron degeneration and stiffness and slowness of the tongue representing upper motor neuron degeneration. This leads to a form of speech disturbance which is difficult to describe but is rather picturesquely described by neurologists as 'hot potato speech'. Very rarely, the first sign of MND is difficulty in breathing due to weakness of the muscles between the ribs which function to expand the chest during normal respiration.

Why are there different names for MND?

A lot of confusion has been generated because neurologists in different countries use different names for the same disease. In the nineteenth century, neurologists recognized that there were some patients who had progressive muscle weakness and wasting due to motor neuron damage. Jean-Martin Charcot in Paris studied the brain and spinal cord of his patients after they had died and noticed that there was evidence of degeneration of the upper and lower motor neurons. He called this pattern **amyotrophic lateral sclerosis** (because there was amyotrophy = muscle wasting and scarring of the connections in the spinal cord that come from the upper motor neurons = lateral sclerosis) and in France and other European countries MND is known as **Maladie de Charcot**. In the USA, MND first came to the attention of the general public when the most famous baseball player in the 1930s developed the disease. In the USA, 'MND' is often known as **Lou Gehrig Disease**. Neurologists in much of the non-USA English-speaking world refer to MND when they mean the broad spectrum of disease patterns described in detail below and reserve the term ALS for the specific form of disease described by Charcot where there is simultaneous upper and lower motor neuron involvement. North American neurologists have adopted 'ALS' as the umbrella term rather than MND. Each term has its merits, and it is largely for historical reasons that both are used.

How do neurologists diagnose MND?

In modern medicine, patients have become used to the idea that doctors have access to an array of sophisticated tests to help guide them towards the diagnosis. For example, the clinical suspicion that a patient is anaemic can be rapidly confirmed by a simple blood test measuring haemoglobin levels. If a patient is suspected of having had a stroke, a brain scan will usually confirm the fact. The role of tests can be overestimated, however. There are many conditions, especially in neurology, for which there are no specific investigations which will establish a definitive diagnosis. Most neurodegenerative diseases are characterized by changes at a microscopic level which do not show up on tests such as magnetic resonance imaging (MRI) scanning. For obvious reasons, we are reluctant to perform a brain biopsy as this would cause more damage. Late on in the illness there may be some evidence of brain shrinkage (known as atrophy), but at the stage when patients are first aware of symptoms and present to a doctor, MRI scanning is generally normal. Similarly, there are no blood tests which can be used to make a diagnosis for diseases such as Parkinson's, Alzheimer's and MND.

MND is a condition in which the process of establishing the diagnosis is referred to as a 'clinical' (from the ancient Greek for 'bedside'). This means that there are no tests which absolutely define MND and it is the opinion of an expert that is the crucial element. Let us now explore how an expert approaches the problem. Typically a patient will be referred to a neurologist, with weakness and loss of function in a limb, or with difficulty with speech and swallowing. The neurologist will listen to the patient's story. If the symptoms have evolved over a period of months and do not obviously involve any other neurological system (e.g. sensation, hearing, vision, co-ordination, etc.) then the neurologist will begin to consider the possibility of a degenerative process affecting the motor system. Physical examination is used to assess the motor system for signs of upper motor neuron damage (stiffness of the limbs, exaggerated reflexes) and lower motor neuron damage (weakness and muscle wasting), but also to verify that the rest of the nervous system is normal. The finding of significant problems with co-ordination of the limbs, with eye movements, sensation or language function, for example, would suggest the possibility of another disease affecting more than just the motor system.

Once the diagnosis of MND has been considered on clinical grounds, most neurologists would then undertake a series of investigations with the aim of excluding more treatable conditions, some of which are discussed below. For example, it is possible that weakness and wasting of the upper limbs combined with stiffness of the lower limbs might be caused by degeneration of the spinal column from ageing and arthritis. Patients with the spinal onset form of ALS therefore require an MRI scan of the spinal cord to exclude the possibility of a degenerative problem that could be treated with an operation.

What sort of investigations are performed in the diagnosis of MND?

It is important to remember that the purpose of the tests outlined below is mostly to exclude other conditions which can be confused with MND. Therefore, depending on the onset and evolution of their disease, most patients will only undergo a few of these tests. On the other hand, it is important, particularly when dealing with such a serious condition as MND, that any doubt about the diagnosis is kept to an absolute minimum. Therefore, tests are sometimes performed even if the likelihood of finding a significant abnormality is very low.

Blood tests

It is always reasonable for a doctor when confronted with a patient with a potentially severe problem to do some blood tests to make sure that there is not a more general health problem affecting many body systems. Such tests will include a **blood count** to look for anaemia and signs of infection, tests of **liver and kidney function** and also **thyroid** hormone status. There have been very rare reports of people with overactive thyroid glands (hyperthyroidism or Grave's disease) who can present with a syndrome of muscle wasting which can look superficially like MND. Therefore, even though the chance of confusion between the two conditions is incredibly low, most patients with MND should have their thyroid gland function checked. When muscle is damaged, an enzyme called **creatine phosphokinase (CPK)** is released into the bloodstream where it can be measured. In situations in which muscle is the primary tissue affected (such as muscular dystrophy or muscle inflammation), the CPK level is greatly elevated (10–100 times the normal value). In MND, where muscle wasting is a secondary consequence of damage to the connecting motor neurons, the CPK level is modestly elevated (up to 2–3 times the normal value). A very high CPK level can therefore sometimes be helpful in alerting neurologists to thinking about other conditions.

Neurophysiological tests

Nerves and muscle are electrically excitable tissues, meaning that they will respond to an electrical stimulus. By stimulating a nerve with a pulse of electricity (in effect a small electric shock!) at one end of a limb and recording the arrival of the electrical pulse at the other end of the limb we can measure how long it takes to travel down a nerve and hence the speed of nerve conduction. In people with MND, the velocity of nerve conduction is normal in surviving nerves. If the conduction velocity in a nerve is reduced, the neurologist would consider other conditions before making a diagnosis of MND. Furthermore, using stimulating needles we can assess the way in which muscle contracts. Normal muscle will give out a little burst of electrical activity when a fine needle is inserted and then it will relax. Muscle that has lost its nerve supply will spontaneously discharge in a pattern that is quite abnormal, even if the muscle itself is not the seat of the problem. Testing muscle in this way is called 'electromyography' (EMG) and allows neurologists to distinguish diseases of muscle from diseases of nerves such as MND. Therefore, most people with a diagnosis of MND will have neurophysiological tests as part of the diagnosis. It should be clear from this discussion that these tests can be helpful in pointing to alternative neurological conditions as well as providing supportive evidence in favour of a diagnosis of MND. It is very important to appreciate that MND begins in a patchy way and therefore sometimes electrical tests are surprisingly normal in patients who have already lost significant function. If all other evidence points towards a diagnosis of MND and electrical tests do not suggest another condition, then an expert neurologist will usually trust their clinical skills and make a diagnosis of MND. An over-reliance on an abnormal EMG as part of the diagnosis can result in considerable delay in having an open and frank discussion between doctor and patient. Of course, as discussed below, there are certainly cases in which it is genuinely difficult to be sure of the diagnosis in the early stages of the disease.

MRI scanning

As explained above, the damage that occurs in MND is at the microscopic level (nerve cells are 1/30 000th of a metre in diameter) and this is beyond the level of detection of current scanning techniques. The main purpose of MRI in suspected cases of MND is therefore to exclude other causes of weakness. A neurologist wishes to know if the neurological abnormality could be caused by a problem in a single location, for example a tumour or a stroke. In most patients with MND, once the disease is past the early stages, the answer is very obviously no, but, as explained above, with such a serious condition it is usually a good idea to do everything in one's power to eliminate any doubt. This sometimes means doing tests when the likelihood that they will alter the clinical diagnosis is very low. Most patients with a diagnosis of MND will have had some form of scanning procedure either to remove all doubt about a treatable condition or, more commonly, because in the early stages there is a genuine possibility that a structural problem in one location could cause the same features.

Lumbar puncture

When the nervous system becomes damaged, various markers of the damage can be found in the cerebrospinal fluid (CSF) which bathes the brain and spinal cord. The function of CSF is partly to cushion the brain against excess movement, but also to provide nutrient support and maintain the correct balance of salts and other chemicals. Examination of the CSF is of most value when the immune system is activated, such as in infections (such as meningitis) or inflammatory conditions such as multiple sclerosis. In MND, the CSF is normal in content and, if the diagnosis is clear, a lumbar puncture is not necessary. Patients who turn out to have MND are more likely to have had a lumbar puncture if their disease pattern is unusual, if they are younger than average or if they do not have early access to an expert in MND.

Is it ever possible that the diagnosis of MND may be incorrect?

Once the disease has developed and takes on its full manifestation, MND is instantly recognizable to neurologists and it only remains for specific tests to rule out the possibility that another disease (such as those described below) might be mimicking MND. However, problems can arise either because patients may be initially referred to a specialist other than a neurologist or quite simply because, in its early stages, MND can be difficult to distinguish from other causes of loss of motor function.

Studies have shown that non-specialists can make errors in diagnosing neurological disease. Up to 30 per cent of patients in one study in which the diagnosis was made by a non-neurologist, did not have MND. Patients who initially have difficulty with speech and swallowing may be referred by their general practitioner (GP) to an Ear, Nose and Throat (ENT) specialist, where the focus may be on excluding a mechanical obstruction to swallowing rather than considering a neurological problem. Older patients who are having difficulty walking may first be seen by general physicians with an interest in diseases of the elderly; in this patient group, the presence of co-existing medical and physical problems (e.g. arthritis) can mask the obvious signs of a neurological disease. When there is weakness of one limb, as often happens first in MND, an Orthopaedic specialist might be asked to investigate the possibility of a 'trapped' nerve root. There are a range of neurological diseases which can affect breathing, and such patients will often be seen by Respiratory Medicine specialists. If any of the above specialists correctly decide that the problem is a neurological one but incorrectly attribute the problem to MND, then mistakes can be made. Particularly in the early phases of MND, when symptoms and signs may be quite restricted, it can sometimes just be difficult to be certain about the diagnosis. Then the neurologist is faced with an apparent dilemma: should the patient be told that a diagnosis is not yet possible or that MND is one of a number of possibilities? We will return to the important area of conveying the diagnosis in a subsequent chapter, but suffice it to say that the diagnostic label of 'MND', once attached, can stick even when the subsequent clinical course suggests that an alternative diagnosis should be considered.

In summary then, for the majority of patients who will have been carefully investigated by a neurologist it is very unlikely that the diagnosis of MND is incorrect. Being certain about the diagnosis, while it can require some painful psychological adjustments, is an important prelude to moving forward and tackling the challenges that MND poses. For this reason, if the patient remains uncertain, most neurologists are only too happy to arrange for a patient with MND to have a second opinion from another colleague.

Which other diseases might be confused with MND?

Patients sometimes tell us that they have encountered stories in the press and on the Internet about patients in whom a diagnosis of MND was initially made but who in reality had another condition. Such stories are given a lot of prominence, which sometimes gives others false hope that another diagnosis will emerge. This can sometimes result in an endless cycle of further tests and opinions. The following is an account of some of the conditions that can occasionally be confused with MND, together with a brief description of how the distinction can be made. This is not designed to turn readers of this book into amateur neurologists, but merely to provide some basic information to help put some of these tales of misdiagnosis into context.

Muscle diseases

Since muscle and nerve work together to achieve movement, it is not surprising that muscle disease can cause weakness. Muscle can be affected by inflammation **(myositis)**, alterations in metabolism (such as **thyroid disease**), genetic conditions such as **muscular dystrophy,** occasionally by degenerative disease **(inclusion body myositis)** or as a side effect of drugs. In general, the pattern of weakness seen in muscle disease is symmetrical and often occurs in a characteristic pattern where muscles closest to the centre of the body (thigh, shoulder, trunk) are affected and the muscles which rotate the eye in different directions are often involved, leading to double vision (something that is never a feature of MND). In addition to these clinical differences, muscle disease can be distinguished from MND by the frequent finding of large (10- to 100-fold) elevations in a muscle enzyme called CPK, which can be measured in blood.

Cerebrovascular disease

Damage to small or large blood vessels from high blood pressure, smoking and cholesterol can sometimes occur in a slow and 'silent' way without an obvious event that is recognizable as a 'stroke'. Damage to the structures in the brain which contain the motor pathways for speech and swallowing can sometimes result in a very similar pattern of bulbar impairment to that seen in MND. Similarly, occasional patients with MND report an apparent sudden onset (they may just be reporting the suddenness with which they noticed the problem rather than its actual onset) which leads to a diagnosis of stroke or 'TIA' (transient ischaemic attack). In most cases, any confusion can be resolved by performing an MRI scan of the brain. However, what happens if a patient develops MND on the background of pre-existing cerebrovascular disease? In this case, the brain scan may well show some damage, but this is incidental. The way things progress usually gives the answer, and electrical tests can help, though with bulbar MND such tests are not always helpful. Given that neurological deficits from cerebrovascular disease are not progressive, time itself can be a most useful diagnostic 'tool', though it may require many months and several clinic visits for uncertainty to be resolved.

Myasthenia gravis

In autoimmune conditions, the normal defence mechanisms in the body used to fight infection and deal with tissue damage can actually cause disease by reacting inappropriately against normal healthy tissue. Myasthenia is an auto-immune condition in which the body produces antibodies which disturb the transmission of signals from nerve to muscle. The weakness that occurs very often produces speech and swallowing disturbance, and can also affect the limbs. As with pure muscle diseases, the weakness is usually symmetrical, affects eye muscles and has the added characteristic of being worse with activ-ity, leading to the complaint of muscle fatigue on exercise. Bulbar myasthenia can be confused with MND, but this is usually resolved using electrical tests of muscle and by looking for the characteristic antibodies of myasthenia in the blood, which are present in the majority of cases.

Benign fasciculations

Because muscle is electrically excitable tissue, it sometimes undergoes spon-taneous contraction. This can manifest either as a cramp or as a flickering known as fasciculation. Most people will have experienced cramps or fascicu-lations after exercise or in cold weather. It turns out that some people, prob-ably because of some inherited genetic variation in the sensitivity of muscle, have very frequent cramps and fasciculation. This is an entirely benign phenomenon which never leads to motor neuron degeneration but, once identified, often does raise concerns that result in referral to a neurologist. It may not surprise you to know that a large number of people who become wor-ried by fasciculations are doctors or medical students! The distinction is made by careful history and examination, and occasionally with the help of EMG.

Degenerative spinal disease

The ageing vertebral column (spine) is highly susceptible to degeneration or 'wear and tear'. Most adults in middle to late life will have evidence on MRI scanning of narrowing of the spaces in the spinal column where nerves exit and travel to the arms and legs and also sometimes the hollow space where the spinal cord itself sits. This can produce compression of nerves and/or the spinal cord, leading to weakness and wasting of muscle in the arms and spasticity of the legs, just like spinal onset MND. The distinction is often clear because the sensory pathways are also affected, but this is not invariably the case, and in suspected cases of spinal onset MND an MRI scan of the spine is usually required to rule out significant structural disease. Because of age-related degenerative changes, MRI scans of the spine are rarely entirely normal in middle-aged and elderly patients, and a careful judgement about the relevance of abnormal findings is required. There is sometimes uncertainty, and some patients will undergo spinal surgery but continue to develop progressive loss of function until it is finally appreciated that MND was in fact the diagnosis from the beginning.

Other motor nerve disorders

This is perhaps the single most difficult and complex area of confusion. MND/ALS is not the only condition that targets motor neurons. There are a large number of genetic diseases in which motor neurons are the principal cell affected. Individually these are rare, but collectively affect a significant number of people. Usually characterized by very slow progression, the onset is often at a younger age compared with MND. Lower motor neuron diseases of this kind are known as **spinal muscular atrophies**. The distinction from MND/ALS is usually clear because weakness and wasting occurs over decades and is very symmetrical, unlike spinal onset MND. Pure upper motor neuron degeneration is known as **spastic paraplegia** and is very often genetically inherited, with over 30 different genetic variants described. The absence of wasting and fasciculation, the symmetrical predominantly lower limb involvement and the presence of a family history usually make the distinction from MND relatively straightforward.

A condition that is not infrequently confused with MND is known as **multifocal motor neuropathy with conduction block**. In this rare disease, the immune system appears to attack nerves to prevent the transmission of the electrical impulse ('conduction block'). This can usually be detected by measuring the speed of nerve conduction. It responds to manipulation of the immune system by regular infusions of immunoglobulin. This treatment has been tried in MND and clearly does not have the same beneficial effect. Another condition that can occasionally be mistaken for MND is known as chronic inflammatory demyelinating polyneuropathy or **CIDP**. It usually has a prominent effect on sensory nerves but, in its rarer, pure motor form, can cause diagnostic confusion. Again, nerve conduction tests are usually very helpful in making the distinction.

What are the different forms of MND?

There is a remarkable degree of variation in the way that MND affects people. This includes variation in the rate of disease progression and also in the regions of the body affected. Descriptions of the disease are usually expressed in terms of the 'average patient', and yet each person with MND is on their own individual journey. It is important that people with MND can remain firmly grounded in what is happening to them and not have to rely on comparisons with other patients who may have a very different pattern of disease. Does this variation in distribution of weakness and the rate of progression suggest that MND is one disease with a very variable course or a series of different diseases with some common features? The answer to this important question is the subject of much research and has not been finally settled, but most experts feel that evidence from post-mortem studies supports the view that the different forms of MND reflect a common pathological process. The brief description of the different terms used to describe MND is given below, and in subsequent chapters we deal with the different patterns of progression seen.

The term **amyotrophic lateral sclerosis (ALS)** was coined by Charcot in the nineteenth century to describe patients with a mixture of wasting and weakness (lower motor neuron degeneration) and stiffness of muscle (upper motor neuron degeneration). This is the most common form of MND and accounts for about 85 per cent of patients. As explained above, it can present with limb weakness ('spinal onset') or difficulty with speech and swallowing ('bulbar onset'). Where bulbar symptoms dominate the clinical picture, the term **progressive bulbar palsy** (PBP) has been used in the past, though it is a term which is less common now. However, within the spectrum of ALS, there is a very wide range of rates of disease progression, so the term is helpful in describing which parts of the nervous system are involved, but in itself does not tell us precisely how the disease will progress. People with ALS do not have one rate of progression.

When there is no evidence of upper motor neuron involvement, MND is referred to as **progressive muscular atrophy** (PMA). About 10 per cent of patients present in this way.

Primary lateral sclerosis is a very unusual form of MND, accounting for approximately 1 per cent of cases, and in which the lower motor neurons in the spinal cord appear to be largely unaffected. Patients present with marked stiffness, usually starting in the legs and ascending over time to involve the arms and the muscles of speech and swallowing. This form of MND can be very slowly progressive and, while it may have a significant impact on mobility and independence, lifespan may be normal.

Regional forms of MND

Some patients attending an MND clinic have a pattern of weakness that can remain confined for very long periods of time to one region of the body. One such pattern is when weakness begins in the legs and progresses only very slowly over several years, leading to loss of walking but with normal function in the arms and other muscles.

2

The cause of motor neuron disease

! Motor neuron disease: key facts

- MND is a neurodegenerative disease which is related to ageing

- So far there has been a lack of useful information from studying the environment and life histories of MND patients

- Genetic studies have identified the cause of MND in a minority of families with inherited disease

- Studies of the abnormal forms of the SOD1 gene suggest that protein accumulation is an important part of the disease process

- Neuropathology has been helpful in distinguishing MND from other diseases and in identifying ubiquitin as a key component of the accumulated protein

- Motor neurons are very long cells which have a specific set of vulnerabilities

---

MND is just one of a group of **neurodegenerative diseases**. These are conditions in which the nervous system develops normally, functions adequately for a period of time (usually many years), but then for some reason fails because specific regions of the brain undergo cell death. As with other medical conditions, neurodegenerative diseases were described and named in an era when little was known of their cause. Neurologists grouped patients together as having a single common disease based on a combination of clinical features (what could be observed by history and examination in life) and pathological features (what could be observed under the microscope after death).

Examples of common neurodegenerative diseases include **Alzheimer's disease** (a progressive loss of memory and language function, but with preservation of muscle power and sensory function) and **Parkinson's disease** (a specific loss of cells in structures deep in the brain which control posture and movement, leading to slowness, tremor and stiffness, but notably without weakness). The cause of age-related neurodegenerative disease is the subject of intensive research efforts. As our understanding of heart disease, stroke and cancer improves and these diseases become treatable and even preventable, an increasingly ageing population makes it likely that neurodegeneration will become the major public health problem of the twenty-first century.

Understanding the progress of current research into MND is important to patients and their families. Many people with MND are motivated to contribute to research, often in the clear knowledge that the benefits of such research may not come for many years. The many strands of research into the causes MND/ALS are discussed and explained in this chapter. In Chapter 7 we consider the implications for individuals with MND of active participation in a research project.

Can studying the pattern of disease in populations give us any clues why people develop MND?

 Epidemiology of MND: key facts

- The probability of developing the disease increases with age

- Although knowledge is incomplete, the incidence of MND appears to be constant throughout the world

- There is currently no evidence to support the belief that MND is becoming more common, except for the expected increase due to greater overall life expectancy

- Men are about one and a half times more likely than women to get MND

- There are no obvious racial factors

- There is only weak evidence at present to suggest that the environment plays a role in determining who gets MND

Understanding the pattern of disease in populations can give important clues as to the cause. This branch of research is known as **epidemiology**. For instance, if a disease occurs in a seasonal or epidemic pattern within defined populations, an infective cause such as a virus is likely. Similarly, in the nineteenth and twentieth centuries many diseases such as chronic lung disease were linked with particular occupations such as mining. Geographical variation in disease patterns may indicate a complex interplay between inherited and environmental factors. For example, when populations from South Asia (India and neighbouring countries) migrate to Europe or the USA and adopt 'Western' dietary habits, there is a marked increase in diabetes and heart disease. This is thought to be because genetic variants which are advantageous in one environment (e.g. where food is scarce) become disadvantageous in another setting (where food is plentiful). Often it is a combination of genetic and environmental factors which can explain epidemiological variation. The classical methods of epidemiology include cohort studies (in which a group of people are followed-up prospectively over many years to see how disease develops), case–control studies (retrospective comparison of risk factor profiles between a group of people with a disease and a group of people acting as normal controls) and investigation of epidemics (an unexpected rise in the incidence of a particular condition).

MND/ALS presents a number of challenges for epidemiologists:

- Its relative rarity means that getting enough patients to study is difficult and requires drawing patients from a large geographical region. This risks failing to identify local environmental exposures which have an effect on small populations.

- A late onset disease may reflect exposures that occurred remotely in time. People are much more geographically mobile than in the past. It may be necessary to take account of where people have lived throughout the whole of their life in order really to understand how environment can be relevant.

- Interest in possible environmental effects is often sparked by clusters of cases. A patient once came to our clinic and showed us a picture of his College football team from 50 years previously. In addition to himself, two other team members had suffered from MND. How can this 'cluster' be explained unless there is something in their shared environment? There are several reasons why cluster analysis has proved unrewarding. First, there is the simple fact that a cluster may be due to chance. If you throw a handful of rice in the air, then it is probable that a few grains of rice among the thousands will land on top of each other. That is to say, truly random distributions do not produce an even geographical separation between cases but inevitably result in a low frequency of apparent clusters. People are not randomly distributed across the land but naturally cluster in towns and villages, further increasing the likelihood of apparent case clusters. Secondly, the identification of clusters leads to an arbitrary definition of the study population. This is often referred to as the 'Texan sharpshooter problem'. The Texan sharpshooter (Fig. 2.1) was a fabled marksman who used to fire his gun randomly at the side of a barn and then proceed to draw the target so that the bullseye was around his hits! In the example given above of the football team, we may be surprised that three out of 12 men in a photograph have developed MND, but what if we considered not just the men in the photograph but all the members of the college as the study population (several hundred), or indeed all of the members of the university (several thousand). The level of significance changes with the chosen denominator population. Rigorous epidemiology requires that the target population is defined before the cluster is identified, not afterwards.

◆ Most cases of MND are studied by neurologists who specialize in the condition and who, by taking an interest in the condition, attract more patients with MND to their clinic. These clinic-based studies are inherently biased because only certain cases (perhaps including a fair proportion of the least typical) are referred. The cumulative 'experience' of one neurological clinic is a highly selective group of cases which may not reflect the pattern of disease as a whole.

In summary, the only really valid forms of epidemiological study for a disease use a **prospective** design (the group of people being studied is identified before

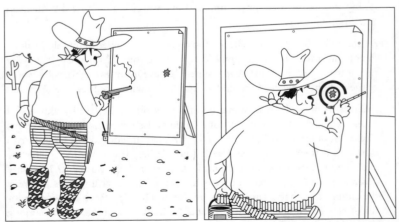

The identification of a cluster and its source population is all too often like the Texan sharpshooter who first fires his bullet and only then draws the target round it.

Figure 2.1 The Texan sharpshooter. Defining the target after we have fired the bullets will always lead to a bullseye!

the disease develops) and are **population based** (there is a clear definition of who is being studied, e.g. the total population of one country or region, with a clear geographical boundary). This presents great logistical difficulties and is a very long-term project. In fact, only a handful of such studies have ever been performed in MND. While these studies indicate that the incidence of MND is broadly the same in each area studied (including Scotland, Southern Italy and Washington State in the USA), these are all populations with predominantly European genetic backgrounds. We know little about the pattern of occurrence of MND in non-European populations, though superficially the disease seems to have very similar characteristics in Japan and India.

It is common sense that our environment (what we eat, where we live, where we work) can influence our health. Changes in diet, activity levels, patterns of smoking behaviour and other 'lifestyle' factors clearly influence the chance of developing ischaemic heart disease. There is a widespread suspicion among many people with MND that their disease may have been caused by some environmental nerve poison. Many different types of substance have been suggested as potentially relevant. For example, certain heavy metals (lead, thallium, mercury, etc.) can be toxic to the nervous system. Similarly, organophosphates used in insecticides such as crop sprays can cause neuromuscular toxicity in overdose. Although the pattern of symptoms and nerve damage from acute toxicity is quite different from that seen in MND, it is legitimate to consider whether low level exposure over many years can be a contributing factor in the development of motor nerve degeneration. However, none of these suspected nerve toxins has yet been shown to be a clear risk factor. Epidemiologists have performed large studies in which they have compared people with MND and a carefully matched control population across a range of risk factors such as occupation, diet and rural versus urban environment. One problem with this approach is that in order to identify a risk factor by asking questions, it is necessary to have a prior assumption about the kind of risk factor to ask about. It is therefore a relatively 'closed' approach which could miss unanticipated associations.

Suggested, but unconfirmed, risk factors for MND

- Exposure to insecticides (organophosphates), employment as a farmer

- Heavy metals (mercury etc.)

- Electromagnetic radiation (from power cables and pylons) and employment as an electrician

19

- Solvent exposure

- Fractures and other trauma

- Athleticism

- Military service (e.g. Gulf War)

Even if it seems a reasonable idea, we cannot assume that all diseases are caused by environmental factors. This has to be proved by careful study. As outlined above, this is very difficult for a disease such as MND but is an important area of continued enquiry. Even though studies performed to date have largely failed to come up with reproducible associations between MND and environmental factors, further study is particularly important in understanding exactly how genes and environment might act together. To this end, several large-scale population studies have been established in Europe and the USA, which over time will be able to answer some of these important questions.

One of the problems with environmental factors which exert very small effects is that it may be difficult to make sense of this in biological terms. For example, even if smoking doubles the risk of MND, because it is a rare disease this will only lead to 1 in 500 of all smokers developing MND as compared with 1 in 1000 of all non-smokers. Compared with the risk of lung cancer, stroke or heart disease from smoking (>80 per cent of smokers will develop one of these conditions), this looks like a very weak biological effect in the context of MND. Does this really give us much of a clue about the cause of MND? Because of the uniform incidence of MND across different populations and environments, some investigators have suggested that the relevant environmental factors are present everywhere. If this is true, it will be a very complicated task to identify such environmental factors and to understand how they could operate to cause disease.

Is MND a genetic disease?

 Genetics of MND: key facts

- Ninety per cent of patients with MND do not have an obvious genetic cause for their disease

- It remains possible that a number of genetic variants act together to produce a risk profile for MND

◆ When there is no family history of MND the likelihood that subsequent generations are at risk is very small

◆ Currently a specific gene has been identified in only a minority of familial cases of MND

◆ When the gene abnormality is known in a family, this allows genetic counselling and testing

◆ Genetic forms of MND, though rare, give us important clues to the way the disease develops

◆ Sporadic MND may be a 'complex genetic disease' in which a number of gene variants interact with other factors to determine individual susceptibility

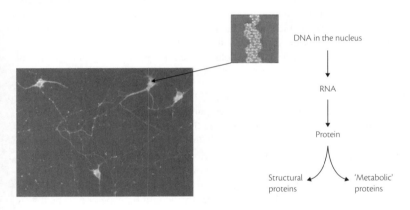

Figure 2.2 Genes control the production of protein in cells. DNA in the nucleus of a cell is used as a template to make RNA, which is then translated into the proteins needed for cell structure and function.

We have approximately 20 000 genes—the same number as a mouse and a chimpanzee! Genes provide the code to produce proteins (Fig. 2.2). Proteins can be the building blocks of cells (analogous to 'bricks and mortar') or the key elements in cell metabolism (energy production, signalling between cells or determining whether cells divide, rest or even die). Given that we are conspicuously different from both mice and chimps, it will be obvious by now that the number of genes does not in itself determine biological complexity.

We now know that individual genes can be processed in a variety of ways such that one gene can give rise to several different forms of the same protein. The way that genes are regulated in humans appears to be more complicated than in other animal species. For example, less than 2 per cent of our DNA actually codes for protein and we appear to have more so-called 'junk DNA' than other species. Although this DNA does not code for protein, it is almost certainly not junk but has important roles in gene regulation. In addition to the differences in gene expression, regulation and processing, proteins themselves are processed differently in different species. The combination of these factors goes some way to explaining why humans are humans and mice are mice. However, we have an awful lot to learn about gene regulation and how different genes interact. Many human diseases are due to mistakes, or *mutations*, in individual genes. In this circumstance, a 'disease gene' can be passed on in a predictable way in families. In other circumstances, a combination of gene variants can predispose to a disease, and because we inherit half of our genes in a random fashion from each parent (like being dealt a hand in a game of cards with 20 000 in the deck), the exact combination that leads to the increased risk only comes together in one member of the family. In this situation, the disease will not be inherited in a simple and predictable way, but could still be due to complex genetic factors. Even with this complex genetic risk profile, there will be additional factors (environmental or just random events which damage cells), which means that only a proportion of people with the risk profile ever develop the disease.

One of the most striking features of MND is that approximately 10 per cent of patients have a clear family history, with the disease occurring in one or more first-degree relatives (parent or sibling) (for a discussion of how MND is inherited in families, see Chapter 6). With common disorders such as stroke or epilepsy, it is not surprising that two closely related family members may be affected for quite different reasons, without having necessarily to explain this by shared genetic factors. Although it is theoretically possible that MND may occur in two family members by chance, this would be expected to be a very rare event indeed. Therefore, when MND is observed in several generations in a single family, this is a strong indication that a specific gene is responsible for the disease. MND which is passed on within an individual family is usually known as **familial ALS** (FALS). Modern molecular genetic methods allow the identification of the location and eventually the identity of a specific gene if it can be tracked through families. A method known as **genetic linkage analysis** uses naturally occurring variations in DNA as markers to identify whether specific DNA markers are inherited with the disease more often than would be expected by chance. Each time DNA is passed on from parent to child, there is a process of 'shuffling' of genetic material called recombination. This ensures that genetic variation occurs and is one of the principal mechanisms driving evolution. Since we know the physical location (i.e. which region of a particular chromosome) of each of the markers, we can infer that a genetic marker that is always inherited by people in the family with the disease, but never by people without the disease, must be very close to the gene causing MND. Genetic linkage studies demonstrate that familial ALS/MND can be caused by defects in a number of different genes.

In the early 1990s scientists tracking the inheritance of MND through families identified mutations in a gene called superoxide dismutase (SOD1). Further work confirmed that about one-fifth of patients with FALS carry mutations in SOD1 (this adds up to about 2–3 per cent of all patients with MND). Identifying a gene for MND was a major breakthrough because, as is explained below, it offers the possibility of understanding what is happening inside motor neurons to make them degenerate. The function of SOD1 is well understood: it is part of the body's system for neutralizing harmful substances known as free radicals, released when cells are under stress. Initially it seemed likely that SOD1 mutations might cause MND by leading to some alteration in the ability of the enzyme to neutralize harmful free radicals. However, there is now a general consensus that in FALS the SOD1 protein causes damage by misfolding and interfering with important functions within motor neurons. Proteins can be understood as a chain of individual building blocks called amino acids, of which there are 20 different types. These small chemical subunits interact with each other to cause the protein to fold into a secondary structure which is determined by the order of the amino acids (the primary structure) (Fig. 2.3).

Some very important questions about how mutant SOD1 causes familial MND/ALS remain to be answered. First, even though FALS is due to a gene abnormality, it still appears to be an age-related disease. People who develop FALS do so with an average age of onset which is about 10 years younger than for sporadic MND. Why can motor neurons tolerate mutant SOD1 for many years before degenerating? The answer is likely to be related to aspects of the way the ageing process affects nerve cells, which therefore provides a common thread linking sporadic and familial MND into the same biological pathways. It must also be the case that motor neurons have some special characteristics which make them more vulnerable than other nerve cells and also cells outside of the nervous system.

Given that most people with MND do not have a simple inherited condition, how can research dissect out the complex genetic factors that might explain susceptibility to sporadic MND? In recent years there has been a rapid increase in our knowledge of the human genome, and several million genetic variants (markers) have been characterized. We now have the tools to analyse these

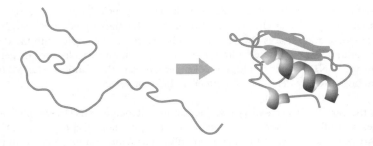

Figure 2.3 Protein folding is critical to their normal function. Proteins exist as a long chain of amino acids which interact with each other according to size and electrical charge. When the protein is allowed to fold it adopts a specific configuration which is an important determinant of its function and interaction with other proteins. It is believed that nerve cells are particularly vulnerable to misfolded protein.

genetic variations at high speed and volume. This kind of 'high throughput screening' allows scientists to test the hypothesis that there are variations in specific genes that occur more frequently in people with MND than in control subjects. However, this approach will only be successful if the genetic variations that predispose to MND are common to most individuals and if a small number of genes exert a relatively strong effect. If a large number of genes exert a small effect in combination, or if many different combinations can lead to the same disease, it will be difficult with current methods to detect this 'signal'. In order to facilitate large-scale genetic screening, a number of collaborative projects are underway to collect DNA from thousands of patients with MND. Within a few years we should have a good idea if this kind of research will reveal how complex genetic interactions might lead to MND and whether it might be possible to predict who is at risk of the disease. It follows that if predictive testing becomes possible, there is the prospect of preventing the disease before it develops.

How do scientists use models to understand the cause of motor neuron degeneration?

The identification of the SOD1 gene as causing a proportion of cases of familial MND has allowed scientists to create model systems in which to try and understand why motor neurons die. Cells grown in the laboratory can be made to produce mutant SOD1 by transferring the DNA encoding the mutant gene for SOD1 into the cell. It turns out that the mutant SOD1 protein forms large aggregations which do not dissolve easily. This appears to have damaging effects on the capacity of cells to tolerate stress such as heat, and inflammation. Because human post-mortem tissue from MND patients has also shown insoluble protein in motor neurons (Fig. 2.4), this has led to the theory that an important part of the cause of MND is a failure of ageing motor neurons to dispose of damaged or mutant protein correctly. Because motor neurons are difficult to grow in the laboratory and also because in the human brain and spinal cord these cells do not exist in isolation but as part of a large network connected to other nerve cells and support cells, there are limitations to what we can learn from looking at isolated cells in a laboratory dish. However, this kind of work provides important preliminary information that can be used to investigate disease processes in whole tissues.

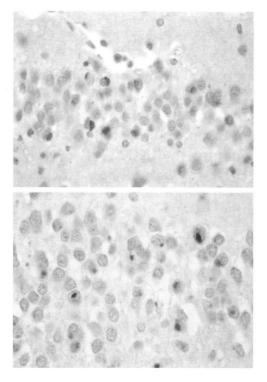

Figure 2.4 Neuropathology of MND. A motor neuron from the brain of a patient who has died of MND shows brown pigmentation which indicates that a protein called ubiquitin is binding to insoluble and misfolded protein within the nerve cell. (Courtesy of Dr Olaf Ansorge, Department of Neuropathology, Oxford Radcliffe Hospital.)

The only realistic way at present to study whole tissues, and therefore an important tool in helping us understand MND is the use of mouse models. It is possible to insert the mutant form of human SOD1 into a mouse embryo so that the adult mouse will express the mutant protein. Such mice do develop motor neuron degeneration that looks superficially similar to human FALS, and they become progressively weak. Many different drugs have been shown to have a positive effect in improving survival in SOD1 mutant mice. Unfortunately, to date, none of the treatments that have shown benefit in mouse models has translated into treatments that work for patients with MND. The reasons for this are likely to be complex but include the fact that laboratory animals are often treated at an earlier stage than would be currently possible in humans. Furthermore, we are still not sure that the pathological processes acting in FALS due to SOD1 mutations are the same as in sporadic ALS. There are very few patients with FALS available to participate in treatment trials, which are therefore always conducted in populations of sporadic MND patients. It must also be acknowledged that the evolutionary gap between mice and humans may simply mean that such a small animal with a short lifespan (approximately 2.5 years) is not a suitable model for human diseases that only develop on average after six decades. However, despite limitations, it is currently the best tool available to us.

What does neuropathology tell us about what is happening in MND?

Doctors who study blood disorders have a distinct advantage over neurologists. The tissue that they are most interested in is very easily accessible just by taking a blood sample or performing a bone marrow biopsy. Because of this, we know a lot about the cause of diseases such as leukaemia, we have ways of monitoring blood diseases and, most importantly, we can replace the cells that are missing or diseased using blood transfusions and bone marrow transplantation. Unfortunately, neurologists cannot biopsy the brain and spinal cord except in very special circumstances as a biopsy would be irreversibly destructive.

Despite this obvious difficulty, we have learned an enormous amount about neurological disease from studying the brains of patients once they have died. In the nineteenth century, when our knowledge of the nervous system was only rudimentary, neuropathology was instrumental in categorizing diseases into groups that seemed to have similar patterns of injury and damage. In this way, we now recognize that different forms of MND are likely to be manifestations of a common pathological process. More recently we have learned that protein accumulation is an important feature of neurodegenerative disease (Fig. 2.4). Pathologists used special techniques to identify the protein accumulating in motor neurons in MND as ubiquitin. The function of ubiquitin is to identify misfolded protein and move it to parts of the cell where it can be processed to prevent it causing harm. The fact that we can see ubiquitin accumulation under the microscope possibly suggests that motor neurons may be damaged in MND because the capacity of the ubiquitin system to handle misfolded protein is exceeded in some individuals. In the future, neuropathology will continue to make a contribution as new molecules and pathways implicated in MND are discovered. It is also possible that we will further refine and classify MND subtypes based on pathological features. It is particularly important that high quality clinical information is accurately matched to pathological data. Brain archives (sometimes referred to as 'Brain Banks') connected closely to an MND specialist clinic have a key role. For information about how to consider brain donation, see Chapter 7.

Can we learn about the cause of MND from brain imaging?

The process of diagnosing MND does not depend on brain imaging, except as a way of excluding other diseases. However, new developments in MRI and other types of scanning raise the possibility that we might be able to track the pathological process in the brain. This would provide new insights into the way that the disease progresses, promote earlier diagnosis and even potentially allow the therapeutic effect of new drugs to be tested on a much smaller sample of people than at present. MRI scanning depends on the fact that hydrogen atoms (in water molecules) can behave like tiny magnets. When biological tissue is subjected to a very strong magnetic field, these little hydrogen magnets all line up in one orientation. When the magnet is switched off, they return to a random orientation and emit a tiny radiofrequency pulse. The pattern of the pulses emitted from the hydrogen atoms in tissue is converted to an image by computer software. The conventional form of MRI scanning creates an image which reflects the structure of the brain and appears as different shades of grey. This is good for identifying brain tumours and other changes in the brain structure, but tells us little about function. If we wish to illuminate the pathways that come from motor neurons and descend into the spinal cord, this is more difficult and requires special computer software to predict statistically which pathways or tracts are travelling together (Fig. 2.5).

Another method, known as PET (positron emission tomography) scanning, involves injecting a tracer (a substance emitting positrons) which travels to the brain attached to glucose and demonstrates changes in regional brain metabolism. Information about changes in the way the brain metabolizes various chemicals which are important for nerve function can provide important clues about neurodegeneration.

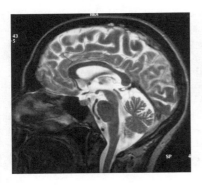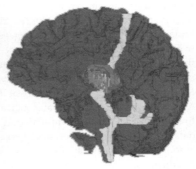

Figure 2.5 Special forms of MRI scanning used in research. **The MRI scan on the left** is a conventional image like those routinely used in hospitals to look for major structural abnormalities. The various shades of grey reflect differences in tissue density, but do not tell us about function. **The image on the right uses** special techniques to highlight regions of the brain in which fibre tracts carrying the projections of nerve cells are damaged in MND.

So far these imaging techniques have tended to confirm what we already know about the areas of the brain affected in MND, which is on the one hand a validation of the techniques but on the other hand has not fundamentally opened any new 'windows' on the nature of the disease. However, this technology is evolving very rapidly and may well be an important part of the contribution to unravelling important aspects of MND pathogenesis.

Why are motor neurons specifically vulnerable to age-related degeneration?

Motor neurons are probably the longest cells in the body. The motor neurons in your spinal cord which travel down your leg to allow you to move your toes are about 1 m in length. The cell body is only 20 millionths of a metre in diameter. This means that a motor neuron is 50 000 times as long as it is wide! The motor neurons in Fig. 2.6 have been removed from the spinal cord of a mouse and grown in the laboratory. If it achieved the actual length it does in humans and was as large as it is in the picture (approximately 1 cm), the end of the cell would be half a kilometre away! It is actually a miracle that such cells survive at all, and there are many mysteries about their function. What is clear is that there must be special transport mechanisms for delivering vital substances such as nutrients down the cell process (called an axon).

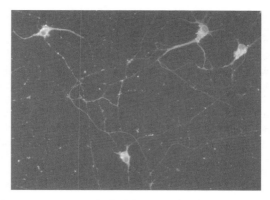

Figure 2.6 Motor neurons grown in the laboratory. This picture gives some idea of the length of the process (axon) of a motor neuron. Proteins have to be transported along the axon in order for the cell to remain healthy.

Axonal transport is one of the most intensively researched areas of motor neuron vulnerability, and there are a number of examples of genetic diseases with some similarities to MND which involve the failure of axonal transport mechanisms.

Motor neurons are also very energetic cells with high metabolic demands. All cells contain small energy-producing 'machines' called mitochondria. Motor neurons are thought to be particularly sensitive to disturbance of mitochondrial function. Both human autopsy material and animal models of SOD1 mutations suggest that mitochondria are among the first parts of the cell to show abnormalities. Drugs that may enhance mitochondrial function have been tried in MND but have not shown beneficial effects, but this is still an area which is the subject of research efforts. A link with ageing may be that as our cells age they accumulate mistakes in mitochondrial DNA.

Another area in which motor neurons may be vulnerable is in their sensitivity to calcium. Nerve cells need chemicals such as calcium, sodium and potassium for many functions including generating the electrical signal to communicate with other nerve cells. However, too much calcium within a cell can be very toxic and triggers cell death. Motor neurons appear to have a reduced capacity to absorb excess calcium. This does not mean, however, that calcium from the diet is harmful, as dietary minerals are very carefully regulated by the body. The elevation of calcium seen in dying motor neurons is more likely to be the consequence of some other cause.

One of the leading theories over the last decade of the cause of MND involves a phenomenon known as excitotoxity. Nerve cells communicate with one another by the release of a small quantity of a chemical called a neurotransmitter (Fig. 2.7). An electrical impulse travels along the axon to the end of a nerve and triggers the release of the neurotransmitter which then activates the next nerve cell. This happens up to many hundreds of times per second in some cells. The most important neurotransmitter activating motor neurons is called glutamate. If cells are overactivated by glutamate, the level of calcium in the cell rises and this is toxic. Some scientists think that motor neurons may be overstimulated in patients with MND, leading to cell death. Why this should happen is not clear. It is possible that it is a consequence of some other pathological process rather than the primary cause. Notably, riluzole, the only treatment which has shown a positive effect on survival, is thought to work by antagonizing glutamate.

What kind of model could explain how MND is caused?

It should now be clear that a range of different processes have been identified as the cause of motor neuron vulnerability. Figure 2.8 is one possible model of how these different elements could combine to cause MND. It should be emphasized that the main elements of this model are still hypothetical. Although these are plausible ideas, with the exception of ageing, we have not yet uncovered clearly reproducible susceptibility factors or disease triggers.

Only when we understand the disease at this fundamental level will be able to design rational treatments to prevent neurodegeneration. This involves a lot of very painstaking fundamental scientific work. Until then, we are left waiting and hoping that a lucky discovery will suddenly give us a vital clue which transforms our understanding of the cause of MND. While this may seem unlikely, in reality science often proceeds by a sudden changes in thinking triggered by a chance discovery. There are numerous examples in the twentieth century, notably the discovery of penicillin by Sir Alexander Fleming. MND research urgently needs such a breakthrough.

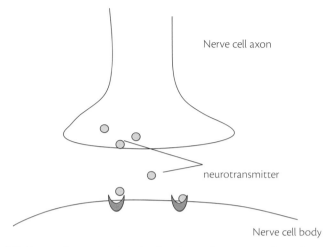

Figure 2.7 Nerve cells communicate by the release of neurotransmitters. Excess amounts of neurotransmitters are thought to overstimulate motor neurons, leading to cell death.

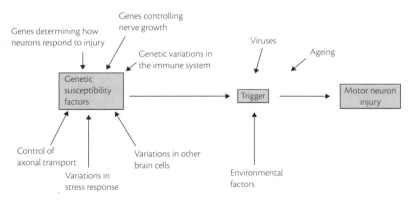

Figure 2.8 What is the cause of MND? The above model is based on the idea that MND develops in people carrying a susceptibility 'profile' in response to an unknown trigger.

3

The individual patient journey

In order to understand how a disease will behave in the long term, doctors often consider their collective experience of looking after hundreds of patients. Questions about how quickly a disease will progress, the anticipated survival time and which functions will become affected with time in different patients can all be answered in this way. However, explanations about the clinical course of MND which refer to 'the average patient' can be extremely unhelpful to an individual living with MND. In reality, MND is a disease which is very variable. It is a fundamental part of our approach to the management of MND to consider the individual patient and their own journey through the disease.

Why is the diagnosis of MND often delayed?

There are several points at which delay in diagnosis can operate (Fig. 3.1). First, the initial symptoms of MND are often very subtle and creep up on people gradually. It is common for people to rationalize minor symptoms as being due to 'trapped nerves', sleeping heavily on a limb, or even simply 'stress'. It is very common to wait until a problem has been present for several months until consulting a GP. At this stage, though the patient is quite clear that the problem is persistent and significant, it may be difficult for a non-neurologist to pick up abnormalities on examination. Many problems seen in general practice resolve spontaneously so, in the absence of clear abnormalities on examination, a period of observation may be required before the significance of a problem can be interpreted. If things become worse, it will be clear to the GP that there is a neurological problem, and a referral is made to a neurologist.

Depending on local variations in access to specialist health care, there may be a delay in seeing a neurologist. Hence many patients have had symptoms for more than 6–12 months by the time they are first seen by a specialist in neurological disease. The first task of the neurologist is to exclude a treatable diagnosis such as the conditions discussed in Chapter 1. This will usually involve an MRI scan and neurophysiological testing as a minimum. This all

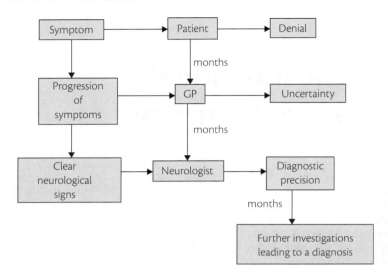

Figure 3.1 The diagnosis of MND is usually delayed. The diagnosis of MND is usually delayed for 1–1.5 years after the first symptoms. This is a combination of the slow onset of the disease, human nature and the absence of a diagnostic test which means that time has to elapse before doctors can be certain that a progressive disease is present.

may take several weeks or months and require a hospital admission. At the end of this process, the neurologist may be certain that MND is the correct diagnosis or there may still be some doubt. Given the severe implications of making a diagnosis of MND, some neurologists still prefer to come to a formal diagnosis only when there is absolutely no doubt. All of these factors combine to explain why the formal diagnosis of MND is often delayed.

We have encountered many patients who are frustrated and angry that it has taken months or years before a diagnosis has been confirmed. While we understand their frustration, the reason in many cases is simply that their disease is progressing at a slower than average rate and has taken a long time to get to the stage where the diagnosis of MND is beyond doubt. This generally indicates a better than average long-term prognosis. We have also met patients who are pleased to be in a specialist clinic setting despite only having had symptoms for weeks or months. Although not always the case, this may reflect a faster than average disease progression.

While the delay in diagnosis can be a source of great frustration to patients and it cannot be denied that avoidable delays sometimes occur, it is also very much a reflection of the nature of the MND disease process. A major priority for research as described in Chapter 2 is to find tests which can promote more rapid and early diagnosis. If we find treatments that slow disease progression, this will become an urgent requirement.

What should a person with MND expect at the time of diagnosis?

It has been demonstrated by research, and is only common sense, that the way in which the diagnosis is conveyed can have a major impact on how an indivual experiences an illness such as MND and can potentially have a lasting influence on psychological well-being. Not so long ago, it was common practice for doctors not to tell the patient when they were suffering from MND, on the grounds that the news would be too distressing or demoralizing and that it was kinder for them to remain in ignorance. This approach, which seems paternalistic and hopelessly naïve by today's standards, left many people only too well aware that something serious was happening to them but without a way to discuss their plight openly. In the modern era, honesty between patient and doctor is an important principle underpinning clinical practice. However, in the early stages, when the full manifestations of the disease may not yet be evident, many neurologists are cautious about using the term MND. While this may leave some people in a 'state of limbo', this caution is motivated by a sincere wish to avoid raising unnecessary anxieties in people for whom MND is only one of a range of possibilities.

The modern Internet age has had an effect in democratizing the flow of information and opening access to knowledge that was previously the preserve of the expert. Therefore, it is unrealistic for doctors to ignore the fact that a patient will come to their own conclusions about what is happening. It is our experience that a spirit of complete openness and honesty is the best way of approaching diagnostic uncertainty. The natural and humane impulse to protect people from distressing information is a positive one. However, research has shown that patients have clear views about what they want from a consultation. Even if the news is bad, patients view a firm diagnosis as a very positive thing. Being left without a clear idea of the nature of a serious illness seems particularly demoralizing.

It is now generally agreed that there are some elements of good practice in conveying the diagnosis. MND should only be diagnosed by someone who is an expert in neurological disease. This is a complicated area, and non-neurologists can make diagnostic errors. The doctor giving the news that some-one has MND must be in a position to support the patient with information, in particular a clear plan for what will happen next. Rapid access to a specialist multidisciplinary team in the early phase is essential. The diagnosis should be discussed in a quiet environment (e.g. a private room not an open ward) without fear of interruption and with plenty of time for questions. As well as the doctor and the patient, it is very important that someone else is present to help support the patient. Ideally this should be their partner or a close relative, not least because that person will also have to absorb the consequences of what is being said. It also helpful to have a second health care professional such as a nurse present. Communicating difficult information is a medical skill which, like any other, will vary from one individual to another. Good doctors understand that people react in very different ways to being given difficult news. The art is to respond to what people want while assuming that most people value complete honesty. It is often helpful to ask the patient what they already know or suspect about the cause of their problem. The initial shock at the diagnosis of MND makes it difficult for people to absorb complex information. The detailed description of MND and its consequences may therefore have to be discussed at a subsequent meeting. Ideally, especially if the diagnosis is made in a hospital ward, there should be an opportunity for a second meeting between the patient and neurologist within a few hours. It is our practice to follow this up with a clinic visit within a few days of the diagnosis. At the first clinic visit we make a tape recording of the consultation, so that the patient can share the information with others of their choosing and also reflect on what has been said. This seems to improve people's experience of a what is inevitably a difficult situation.

The Motor Neuron Disease Association (MNDA) have produced guidelines for best practice in investigating possible MND and in conveying the diagnosis (see Chapter 10).

How do people with MND respond to the diagnosis?

On an individual level the person with MND undergoes a very real bereavement process with a strong sense of personal loss for an anticipated future. Even in the more slowly progressive forms of MND, where coming to terms with a terminal illness may not be uppermost in people's minds, there will still be a sense of loss associated with giving up work, hobbies, travel and other things which most people take for granted.

Psychologists recognize a number of stages in the process of bereavement when someone close to us dies. The same emotions are equally applicable to coming to terms with a diagnosis of MND. The natural stages of bereavement are detailed below.

Shock

A sense of disbelief is common. Why me? The apparent randomness of MND can be a source of difficulty for people. If there is a clear explanation as to why something happens, we usually find it easier to absorb. The bad news that there is something seriously wrong, followed by an admission by specialists that we do not know why it has happened, tends to increase the sense of powerlessness felt by people with MND. The feeling of shock diminishes with time.

Denial

A period of feeling that this all must be a terrible mistake is also a frequent experience for newly diagnosed patients. At this stage, it can be helpful to have a second opinion. Perhaps more common than denial about the actual diagnosis is a failure to accept that there is no cure. This can lead to an endless search for possible treatments on the Internet where there are numerous claims made by unscientific or unscrupulous people that various unproven remedies will cure MND. For a discussion of the hazards of unproven therapies, see Chapter 5.

Anger

Given the devastating nature of MND, a feeling of anger seems an entirely reasonable and rational response. Sometimes anger is directed at health care professionals either because they are the bearers of bad news or because they are perceived to be at fault for not having treatments that work. Anger can also be directed at close family and friends, simply because they are the closest in proximity at a time of stress and trauma.

Guilt

Occasionally people with MND are under the mistaken assumption that they have brought the illness upon themselves, for example by overwork or because they have not coped well with stress, or because of their occupation. It is an important part of the MND specialist's role to reassure people that, as far as we know at present, lifestyle factors are not relevant to MND causation. As indicated above, the random nature of the disease also creates psychological issues. In addition, guilt can affect people once they realize that their own illness inevitably creates a challenge for other people around them. Although it is our general experience that immediate family members show remarkably little resentment towards the person with MND, this can be difficult for patients to appreciate and the guilt feeling can be a considerable psychological burden.

Depression

In many ways it is remarkable that people with MND seem not to get depressed as often as one would expect. While this is a difficult area to study and individual anecdotal experience is unreliable, there is a feeling among specialists that people with MND become depressed far less frequently than other patients with chronic neurological disability, such as multiple sclerosis (MS). There may be specific biological reasons why MS patients experience mood disturbance related to the involvement of brain regions associated with emotion. Whatever the explanation, we have seldom had reason to treat MND patients with antidepressants. However, some susceptible individuals who develop major mood disturbance during the course of MND will certainly benefit from antidepressant treatments.

Acceptance

A natural resolution usually follows these individual stages of bereavement in the vast majority of people with MND. This is an important part of the process of moving forward and engaging in decision making which can increase the individual's sense of control over their situation.

Once the diagnosis is made, what happens next?

People with a diagnosis of MND should have access to a team of health care professionals with knowledge and experience in the management of complex neurological disability. Most people with difficult and relatively rare diseases value the opportunity to talk to experts in the condition. Therefore, an appointment with a neurologist specializing in MND in a regional neuroscience centre is usually viewed as a very reasonable request by GPs and general neurologists. In the UK, a number of neurology clinics, with support from the MNDA, act as Care Centres to provide specialist services for patients with MND (see Chapter 10). Some patients continue follow-up at these centres throughout the whole duration of the illness, while others may make only one visit for advice and information early in the disease. In some areas, MND is managed by specialists in neurological rehabilitation or palliative care. What matters most is that patients have access to people who are interested in their problems and have the expertise to help them.

How often patients are seen in clinic will vary according to individual practice, the rate of change of the disease and personal preference. In general, for typical MND, it is usual for patients to be seen once every 3–4 months. If it becomes clear that the pattern of disease is slower than average, a 6- or even 12-monthly appointment may be appropriate. It is important that appointments are flexible so that unanticipated problems can be dealt with without delay. Between clinics contact by telephone or e-mail should be freely available.

What happens in the MND clinic?

Clinics vary according to the resources available and the style of individual specialists. Here we briefly outline the general structure of MND care in a typical clinic according to the different roles of individual team members. The management of individual symptoms is dealt with in more detail in Chapters 4 and 5. One of the main functions of a multidisciplinary clinic is to provide a single location for co-ordination of all of an individuals needs and to avoid the duplication that can otherwise occur. We recognize that the traditional hospital-based clinic where patients are only likely to meet the doctor are not well suited to the management of a complex condition like MND. Medical expertise is only one of a range of skills that should be available.

What is a multidisciplinary care team?

Owing to the complex nature of MND and the fact that so many things can happen at once, it would be impossible for one person to have all the skills and knowledge to deal with every aspect of the disease. Therefore, a team approach is the best way to ensure that all issues of care are considered. None of the professionals in the multidisciplinary team work in isolation. They may well overlap slightly when looking at one issue; for example, when looking at the nutritional intake of a person living with MND, the dietician and the speech and language therapist (SALT) will work closely together and will also communicate with the neurologist and specialist nurses. The following health care professionals may be involved with the care of a person living with MND:

The neurologist has expertise in the diagnosis and management of MND and in many cases is also likely to have a significant research interest in the condition. In a clinic setting the neurologist is usually the team leader and will take overall responsibility for major management decisions. At the first visit the emphasis will be on reviewing the diagnosis, if made elsewhere, by taking a history of the patient's problem and then performing a physical examination. At subsequent visits, progress will be assessed, new symptoms discussed and questions about research and treatments explored.

The specialist nurse has a great deal of experience looking after people living with MND and will understand the complexities of the disease. The nurse will often be the central co-ordinator of the multidisciplinary care team, particularly within the context of a large clinic such as one of the MNDA-funded care centres in the UK. Specialist neurological nurses are also often attached to Neurology Departments in general hospitals, and some areas may have community-based specialist nurses. Between clinics, they are able to offer ongoing assessment, monitoring and advice, and to involve other members of the team at the appropriate time.

District Nurses are based in the community and are attached to a general practice. They could be involved in the management of MND at any time in the illness, but most commonly they will be involved with people once they have had a percutaneous endoscopic gastrostomy (PEG), or in dealing with issues of continence, the provision of pressure-relieving mattresses and in symptom control in terminal care.

A palliative care team consists of doctors and nurses and other therapists who are expert in symptom control. They work closely with District Nurses, GPs and hospital specialists to bring their particular skills to bear on some of the problems encountered in MND. It is not widely appreciated that a palliative care team can often become involved with people with MND at an early stage and do not just deal with care at the end of life. Similarly, while they are usually based within a local hospice, much of their work is with people in their own homes.

Specialists in respiratory care, both doctors and nurse specialists, are increasingly working as part of the MND care team. They carry out breathing assessments and initiate programmes of care, including non-invasive ventilation, to relieve symptoms associated with breathing muscle weakness.

Occupational therapists (OTs) are based both in acute hospitals and in the community. Occupational therapy is the assessment and treatment of both physical and psychiatric conditions using specific, purposeful activity to prevent disability and promote independent function in all aspects of daily life. They may visit people living with MND at home to monitor their progress, initially assessing function in carrying out day to day activities. Maximizing mobility is particularly important. OTs will supply pieces of equipment such as commodes, toilet seats, bathing aids, grab rails and hoists to help lift people, and advise on adaptations to the home. They may also explain about the Disabled Facilities Grant (DFG) to anyone with a permanent and substantial disability.

Physiotherapy. Many people living with MND benefit from seeing a physiotherapist. The aim of physiotherapy is to maximize independence and prevent secondary disability (e.g. joint stiffness and contractures arising because a limb can no longer be moved through its full range). This might be achieved by establishing an exercise programme that can be performed independently or with the help of carers, or by specific sessions of physiotherapy targeted at a particular area of the body. For people living with MND this will involve stretching exercises. It may also include walking or swimming. Physiotherapists are also able to teach breathing exercises and assisted cough techniques. It will usually be the physiotherapist who supplies equipment such as walking sticks, crutches, walking frames and various splints

Speech and language therapist (SALT). Many people with bulbar onset MND may well have met a SALT at an early stage, even before they have been diagnosed as having MND. The SALT will assist in the differential diagnosis and liaise between specialities such as ENT and Neurology. The SALT works closely with the multidisciplinary team, particularly the dietician, to monitor and advise on problems with speech and swallowing and in the timing of a PEG tube.

The **dietician** has an important role to play in the maintenance of well-being by ensuring that an adequate diet is maintained. This may involve providing samples of different supplement drinks, talking about likes and dislikes, and discussing the whole range of options available to the person living with MND.

Psychology services have a number of roles within the care team. As mentioned in Chapter 6, some patients with MND experience cognitive impairment. Differentiation from depression may require a formal psychological assessment. Psychologists can also help with the management of severe adjustment reactions and anxiety symptoms, or simply provide supportive counselling.

Social and health care managers work with people living with MND and their families to create a plan of care that meets the needs of the individual client. This will include advising about statutory benefits, paying for adaptations to the home and co-ordinating community support.

How will MND progress?

Throughout this book we emphasize the variation in how MND progresses. Overall this can provide some comfort to people whose first impressions of the disease are dominated by the worst aspects. Our message to patients is that MND is a personal journey, and it can be very misleading to draw assumptions about how things will progress from other people's stories. It is not uncommon for unusual cases to get the most publicity. In an effort to offer a simple explanation of the nature of MND, doctors and sources of information such as books and websites, usually describe a 'typical case' and almost invariably all of the possible manifestations of MND are mixed in together. Therefore, patients often arrive in our clinic with a view of the disease which does not fit their own personal circumstances.

It is of course inescapable that MND, being a disease of muscle weakness, can lead to significant and sometimes total paralysis. However, it is not uncommon for patients to go through the whole duration of their illness and retain significant limb strength. We have had many patients who remain able to walk for a significant proportion of the total disease course. Similarly, communication difficulties due to involvement of the muscles of speech may only affect a proportion of patients. The key message is that, without discussion with the specialist MND team, do not assume that any clinical feature of the disease is an inevitability.

When attempting to understand the factors that dictate the prognosis of MND, specialists have studied large groups of patients and drawn generalizations. The challenge, in counselling individuals about their own prognosis, is to apply information derived from these large groups to individuals. In fact it is often very difficult at the first visit to be precise about how the disease will progress, and there are usually a range of possibilities for the future. Even where there are features of MND which are usually associated with a short or long illness duration, there will be some cases which are 'exceptions to the rule', meaning that caution has to be exercised and that time is an important aid to the process of prognostication. However, some broad generalizations, if applied carefully to individuals, can be used to predict how the disease will progress. It turns out, perhaps unsurprisingly, that the speed at which things are changing is a robust indicator of the overall prognosis. If there is only very slow change in the first year (e.g. if weakness remains confined to one limb only) then the prognosis is clearly better than for a patient who has had a rapid progression of disability so that they lose the ability to walk within the first year. This is only common sense but underlines a very important principle: that the pace of change in MND is the same throughout the whole duration of the illness. This is explored further below. Another feature which tends to be associated with a poorer prognosis is early involvement of the muscles of breathing. Again this should be obvious since the reason that MND affects lifespan is chiefly related to the development of respiratory failure. This does not mean that every patient with respiratory muscle involvement automatically has a poor prognosis. We have had a number of patients who have selective involvement of the diaphragm and otherwise slowly progressive disease, who survive for much longer than average. Age can play a role in dictating the overall impact of the disease. For some reason, younger onset patients overall have a slightly slower disease progression than average. At the other end of the spectrum, MND consistently runs a shorter course in the very elderly, probably in most cases due to the co-existence of other medical problems and general frailty. The pattern of disease progression clearly has some influence. When upper motor neurons are the predominant cell involved, the disease runs a much longer course. A similar but less consistent effect is also observed with lower motor neuron predominant MND. Bulbar onset disease is on average associated with a worse prognosis because there is frequently associated respiratory muscle involvement and because weakness of the throat muscles makes people vulnerable to chest infections. All of the above features must be taken together within the context of an individual pattern of MND and speed of progression before deciding the overall prognosis.

The mean survival with MND is quoted in different ways depending on whether it is taken from the onset of symptoms (something about which it is difficult to be precise) or presentation to a neurologist (dependent on many factors, some of which are non-medical such as waiting times for specialist clinics). It is therefore not surprising that different studies give different figures. A reasonable estimate is that approximately 50 per cent of patients with MND succumb to their illness within 2.5 years after onset. As can be seen from Fig. 3.2, approximately

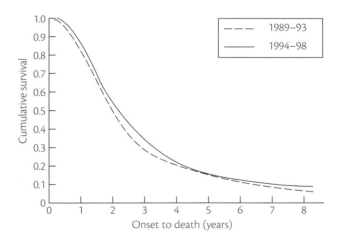

Figure 3.2 Survival rates for MND patients in a population register. Data from the Scottish Motor Neuron Disease Register showing the proportion of people alive at different times after onset. It can also be seen that there is very little difference in the survival rates over time.

one-fifth of patients are still living with MND 5 years after onset. Attempts to study long-term survivors have come up with very few solid conclusions as to why this group fares better. It seems to be simply that in each person the disease is progressing at an individual rate that determines the total duration.

Can MND speed up or slow down, or even stop progressing?

The rate at which the process of neurodegeneration occurs is thought to be the same throughout the whole duration of the illness. This leads to a clinical progression rate which is steady. However, patients with MND sometimes report that they feel that the disease has changed its rate of progression for a period of time, either entering a plateau phase where not much seems to change for a long time, or appearing to speed up. In the clinic we observe the disease closely by reviewing patients on a regular basis, usually every 3–4 months. For the majority of patients with typical MND, there are measurable changes at each clinic visit. However, there are undoubtedly atypical patients in whom the rate of progression is so slow that it is really very difficult to discern any change at each clinic visit. We do not think this is because the disease has genuinely stopped progressing, however. Similarly, some people with MND are firm in their view, despite what we say about the rate of progression, that their illness has proceeded more rapidly than expected in the interval between clinics. The way to understand this is to consider that a complex function such as walking requires many different muscle groups to act together. As the muscles acting around joints such as the hip, knee and ankle become weak, other muscles will attempt to compensate, tending to preserve function. A point will come when this compensation breaks down, producing a sudden 'milestone' such as losing the ability to walk. Although this appears to have happened abruptly, it is really a steady process that has manifest rather suddenly because of a breakdown of compensatory muscle function.

How can people with MND cope as the disease progresses?

In the clinic we find that there is a tension between the natural human tendency to 'live for today', ignoring what may happen tomorrow, and the need to look ahead so that plans can be made. We often encourage people to try and deal with the future by thinking in meaningful timeframes. For each individual, the pace of change of their disability will dictate whether the appropriate timeframe is a few months or longer. What matters is that change is anticipated and plans are made to accommodate a change in function.

While the wish to suppress difficult thoughts about what will happen in the future is natural—'I will worry about that when it happens'—this generally leads to crisis management and frantic attempts to catch up with a changing set of circumstances. Particularly for people who live alone, this can lead to a loss of control over personal circumstances. Clear and frank discussion of the challenges that MND poses for people living with the disease can give back some control, in a situation in which the disease often seems to be dictating events. In Chapter 8 we discuss in detail how people with MND can confront decisions at each stage of their disease.

4

The treatment of motor neuron disease and the management of specific symptoms

Introduction

MND is not currently a curable disease, and many patients report having felt abandoned by doctors, who may appear uncomfortable with a patient whom they believe they cannot help. In reality, there are very few diseases which are genuinely curable, and most doctors are engaged in managing chronic symptoms, rather than simply 'curing' people. Like many other conditions in medicine, MND also has specific symptoms which can be managed. The overall aim of this approach is to focus on maintaining well-being. As we have highlighted elsewhere, the range of symptoms and problems encountered in MND is best managed by a multidisciplinary team in a centre in which MND patients are seen on a regular basis.

Have clinical trials demonstrated that there are drugs which can slow the progress of MND?

There is now an intensive research effort to identify drugs which can slow down the process of motor neuron loss, arrest the progression of disability and improve survival in MND. Drugs are usually selected on the basis that they have shown an effect in a model system (such as the SOD1 mouse described in Chapter 2) or in another neurodegenerative disease. New drugs receive a licence for use in a particular disease if an effect has been shown in a carefully conducted clinical trial. This process is described in Chapter 7. A large number of drugs, with plausible mechanisms of action that might modify neurodegenerative disease, have been tried in MND. In recent years these trials have been conducted to a relatively high standard and we can be confident that we have not missed a useful treatment effect. What is not clear is whether combinations of drugs might have an effect where single agents do not. Developments in the field of cancer treatment have taught us that several drugs used in combination can be effective where individual drugs in isolation are not. Given that there is good experimental evidence that a number of different pathways are involved in the death of motor neurons, it is reasonable to suppose that combination drug therapy would be a good strategy in MND. Unfortunately, unless we are looking at large effects on disease progression, it is very challenging to find ways to conduct clinical trials of multiple agents in combination in a relatively rare disease. Very few trials of drug combinations have been performed in MND. One exception is the combination of riluzole and vitamin E, but this did not show an enhanced effect over riluzole alone.

Should I be taking riluzole?

To date, only riluzole (marketed as Rilutek™) has shown any effect on survival, and there is still some debate about its true benefit. The rationale for trying riluzole is that it antagonizes the effect of a neurotransmitter called glutamate (see Chapter 2). Excess glutamate has been implicated in the death of motor neurons in MND. Cumulative evidence from several clinical trials in which riluzole was given to almost 900 patients, and compared with over 400 patients given placebo, demonstrated a small effect with riluzole in prolonging survival. This is often quoted as amounting to 2–3 extra months of life with MND. It is important to appreciate that the only plausible effect that riluzole could exert on the disease is to slow the progress of motor neuron loss. Therefore, functional deterioration will still occur, but hopefully more slowly. There are no expected effects in improving muscle strength or in alleviating any of the symptoms of MND. However, there are many unanswered questions. Do all people benefit equally? Is there more benefit if the drug is given very early in the disease? Are elderly people with MND likely to benefit as much as younger people (clinical trials usually restrict entry to the under 75 age group)? If riluzole prolongs life by several months in people with typical ALS-type MND, does that mean that people with more slowly progressive forms of disease should expect commensurate increases in survival, even extending to several years in some cases? After more than a decade of experience, most specialists agree that the effect of riluzole is likely to be modest. Comparisons of current groups of patients with those from the past, although made difficult by the complex changes in the delivery of care to people with MND that have occurred in the last 10 years, have not demonstrated clearly that, even with the widespread availability of riluzole, people with MND are living longer overall. However, it is currently the only therapy licensed for the treatment of MND, and most patients feel strongly that is should be available, indicating that even if the effect is modest it is considered meaningful by those living with the disease. Generally the side effects of riluzole are minor. About 1 in 10 people given the drug do not tolerate it because of lethargy or gastrointestinal disturbance (nausea and vomiting). In this respect it compares well with most drugs used in medical treatment, so taken in a general context it should not be considered to be a hazardous drug. Generally, we find that the elderly age group are more susceptible to adverse effects so we are more cautious in using riluzole in this group. Because it can lead to a rise in liver enzyme activity (which is not always a sign that the liver is actually damaged), it is necessary to check liver function with blood tests every month for the first 3 months and then every 3 months for the first year of treatment.

Despite the apparent modest effect on survival with riluzole, in our experience a significant number of patients elect not to take it. Some people feel that they do not wish to prolong the course of their disease if there is no effect on quality of life. Others, who have studied the evidence for themselves, just conclude that the benefits are too modest to justify taking a tablet every day. Some people are worried about side effects. What matters overall is that people with MND have the opportunity to receive expert help in making an informed choice.

What about drugs for which there is not yet evidence?

Most people understand that drugs have to be subjected to clinical trials before they can be used safely. However, people living with MND are understandably frustrated by the slow pace at which drugs that appear to show benefit in research experiments are applied to the treatment of patients in the clinic. Some of these drugs are already licensed for use in other conditions and therefore could be prescribed to patients with MND as a so-called 'off-licence' prescription. People with MND have every right to feel that time is running out for them and that they cannot wait for the kind of evidence that would satisfy doctors. What do we advise people to do in this situation? It is important to be realistic and to realize that, to date, of all of the drugs that have shown some kind of promise in trials in animal models, riluzole is still the only one which has demonstrated any kind of benefit in human MND. Therefore, it is on balance unlikely that today's patients are missing out on a therapy that will transform their situation. All drugs have side effects, and taking combinations of substances inevitably increases the probability of an adverse reaction. When patients with MND ask our advice whether they should take medicines for which there is currently no evidence of benefit, we are ethically bound to point out that we have no evidence to support recommending this. However, we fully understand why some people choose to take speculative therapies and, as long as there is no clear evidence of significant harm and medical supervision is maintained, a case can sometimes be made. The following are examples of substances that are taken by patients with MND for which there is either no evidence of benefit or even good evidence of lack of benefit.

◆ There is theoretical evidence that **vitamin E**, an antioxidant, protects degenerating nerve cells. It has been tried in various diseases such as Alzheimer's, Parkinson's and MND. None of these trials has shown an obvious benefit. It remains possible that it could still have some sort of effect. It is not harmful and it can be obtained easily from pharmacists without a prescription. Very high-dose vitamin E (so called 'megadose therapy' of up to 5000 mg per day, which is many hundreds of times the normal dietary intake) is equally speculative but does carry potential side effects (usually moderate gastrointestinal symptoms such as nausea/diarrhoea) and requires a prescription.

◆ **Minocycline**. This is an antibiotic which is available on prescription. There is evidence from animal experiments that it may slow down the course of MND. At the time of writing, human trials are in progress.

◆ **Creatine**. This is used by bodybuilders. It may generally enhance muscle performance. It has been tried in MND but did not show any effect on survival or on function. The doses used were 5–10 g per day. It is not generally recommended by most MND specialists, but is freely available in pharmacies.

What is the role of alternative or complementary therapies in MND?

We understand that patients with MND wish to do everything that they can to remain well and to slow down the disease process. Health care professionals should adopt a non-judgemental approach and view their role as providing information. It is preferable for doctors seeing people with MND to know if their patients are being treated by practitioners outside mainstream medicine as it helps them understand individual beliefs about health and illness and put other available treatments in context. Modern medical practice is underpinned by the belief that we have an ethical responsibility first to offer treatment for which there is proven benefit from clinical trials and, secondly, to do no harm. Many patients seek help from 'alternative' or 'complementary' practitioners. The definition of 'alternative' is not precise, but the following are some of the ways in which the term is used.

◆ Any treatment which is outside of 'conventional' medicine as practised by doctors in hospitals. This is a reasonable factual definition.

◆ Something which is 'natural' and therefore not harmful, in contrast to conventional therapies which are seen as 'artificial' and by implication harmful. However, it is important to appreciate that many of the most important drugs in use in hospitals today (especially antibiotics and anti-cancer drugs) come from plants. There are also numerous examples of so-called natural remedies being associated with harmful and even fatal adverse effects.

◆ Something which works in a fundamentally different way from normal treatments and to which it would therefore be inappropriate to apply the same standards of evidence in deciding a beneficial effect. An example of this might be faith healing or the power of prayer. Practitioners who take the view that they do not need to provide evidence of benefit (or at least evidence of lack of harm) are therefore acting differently from conventional medical doctors, because they claim benefit for their treatments without providing evidence. Although within the framework of a scientific culture, this might be viewed as unethical, it could be entirely consistent with a spiritual belief system.

Neurologists specializing in MND have no fixed or blinkered view about what might work in preventing progression in MND. We believe that all therapies, whether deemed conventional or alternative, should be studied in the same way. The distinction between conventional and alternative could more usefully be replaced by:

◆ **'treatments that are effective'**: this could easily include effectiveness in providing emotional and spiritual help as well as physical benefit

◆ **'treatments that are ineffective'**

◆ **'treatments that are harmful'**: this could include physical harm if there are adverse side effects, financial harm if they are expensive, and mental harm if they involve giving false hope through deception.

It is, of course, possible for treatments to be both simultaneously effective and potentially harmful or, worse, ineffective and harmful. There are practitioners both in the UK and abroad encouraging patients with MND to try treatments for which there is no evidence of benefit. In many cases, this does little harm.

In other cases, there are serious concerns that vulnerable individuals are being misled into paying large sums of money and also exposing themselves to risk. We would strongly advise people with MND to discuss each treatment that they are contemplating with their MND clinic specialists. Examples of treatments which do not seem harmful but for which there is no specific evidence of benefit include acupuncture, massage, reflexology and homeopathy. Examples of treatments for which there is no evidence of benefit but which could be harmful (even just by being uncomfortable or very expensive) include chelation therapy, exclusion diets, taking any combination of unidentified herbs, chemicals, powders or extracts, and removal of dental fillings.

 Patient's perspective

Derek is a 55-year-old farmer with spinal onset MND. Six months after we first began seeing Derek in clinic we were contacted by his brother who was very concerned that Derek seemed to be spending large sums of money on some form of 'herbal powder' that he was purchasing from a private doctor. Derek's brother was especially worried because he knew that Derek was not a wealthy man and that he had borrowed the money from his elderly parents who had offered him their life savings in the hope of getting help. At the next clinic visit we asked Derek about other treatments he was receiving. He told us about the 'natural medicine clinic' he was attending and that the doctor there had told him that he could cure MND using a 'holistic approach'. Derek had been given a brown powder to take every day, which cost £200 per month. The doctor in the clinic had referred Derek on to other clinics and he had undergone a range of other treatments. We explained that there was no evidence that such herbal powders could treat MND. He explained that we said we couldn't cure him and that he had found someone who said that he could, so he wanted to give himself the chance. Derek died of MND 2 years after onset, leaving debts of £16 000.

Ideally, the patient and doctor act in a partnership based upon mutual trust, and the benefit of any treatment should outweigh the likely risk. People who are suffering from diseases for which modern medicine does not have many answers are particularly vulnerable to deception from those who make exaggerated claims. The Internet is a great force for democratization and for increasing access to specialist information. However, it is not always clear to the non-expert whether information offered on the Internet is valid. There are few data on how many people with MND seek help from alternative or complementary practitioners. Our experience is that this is common, but patients who seek such help may not feel able to admit this to mainstream doctors. In one study from Germany which looked at the use of alternative therapies in MND, approximately 50 per cent of all patients were consulting either a homoeopathist, a naturopath or some other form of alternative therapist, and these patients spent on average several thousand Euros on such therapies. Interestingly, the study suggested that the people who took up such therapeutic options were the ones who were most enthusiastic about conventional therapies and inclusion in drug trials. Therefore, it may be that the use of alternative therapies by people with MND is a feature of the patient who wants to do everything they can to slow their disease down. This is of course a very positive form of behaviour. Even if the exaggerated claims made about various treatments are made in 'good faith', not with deception, the harm that they cause is still an injustice for the individual who is affected. Of course, many of these treatments are practised by people with the best of intentions, who do not seek to deceive those that they treat and who may even, despite the lack of formal evidence, make people feel better. We have had many patients who have told us that they found it helpful or comforting to have treatment from a faith healer or herbalist. When alternative treatments do not cause harm and are offered as a way to improve well-being without any exaggerated claims for their effect on the course of the disease, we accept that this may improve a patient's experience of their illness.

How does MND lead to weight loss?

The most obvious reason why people with MND may lose weight is the simple fact that muscle mass is lost through atrophy. While this may simply be a consequence of motor neuron degeneration, some scientists think that an alteration in muscle metabolism occurs in some people with MND.

Eating and drinking are central to our domestic and social life. There are very few social events which do not include refreshments of some sort. Therefore, if eating becomes more difficult it can have a devastating effect, both emotionally and physically. However, it is an area in which a great deal can be done to restore and maintain well-being, provided a step by step approach is taken and interventions are timely. Depending on the pattern of MND, the muscles involved in chewing and swallowing can become slower, stiffer and weaker in various combinations. People with bulbar onset MND are likely to experience these problems at an earlier stage than those with spinal onset MND. However, it is important to note that some people may never actually experience significant swallowing problems at any time in the illness. To understand why eating and drinking can become difficult, it is important to have some idea of normal swallowing (Fig. 4.1). Part of the act of swallowing is under voluntary control, but much of the swallow is an involuntary or reflex action. Swallowing involves the lips, cheeks tongue, jaw, oesophagus and epiglottis.

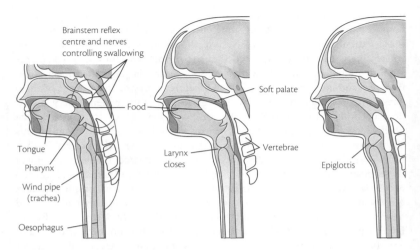

Figure 4.1 The swallowing mechanism. Normal swallowing involves the co-ordination of the lips and tongue (voluntary muscles) with the palate and throat (involuntary muscles) to produce the swallowing reflex.

When we take food into our mouths, the lips act as sensors detecting heat and directing food to be chewed using the teeth, and muscles in the cheeks and jaw. The saliva in the mouth helps to soften the food and starts to aid the breakdown of the food particles. Swallowing problems therefore begin in the mouth, with weak lips preventing good closure (lip seal), jaw weakness preventing adequate chewing and difficulty with the tongue manoeuvring the food bolus into a good position for swallowing. Food may also collect under the tongue.

Once the food has been formed into a ball (bolus) of food it is moved to the back of the throat by raising the tongue to the roof of the mouth. The muscles of the throat contract and squeeze the food over the tongue towards the oesophagus (the tube which transports the food to the stomach). As the food reaches the oesophagus the larynx (voice box) rises up and closes, and the epiglottis closes over the trachea (wind pipe). The muscles of the oesophagus then relax and the food is pushed down towards the stomach. Because this is such a complicated process, it does not take a great deal of change in the muscles to result in significant problems. A sensation that swallowing is difficult is called **dysphagia**. Food arriving in the oesophagus before the epiglottis has had a chance to close can result in an uncoordinated swallow causing coughing or the sensation of choking, leading to a genuine fear of eating. Despite our experience that people with MND do not suffer a major medical mishap during choking fits, it can be a frightening experience and it can be difficult to provide reassurance. Another concern is that tiny fragments of food enter the lung and may cause infection.

If eating and drinking become difficult, one obvious consequence is that intake is inadequate to meet daily needs. However, equally important for well-being is that mealtimes are no longer a pleasure, opportunities for social interaction are lost, meals take longer, food becomes unappealing because it may become cold, and a vicious cycle is established where mealtimes are surrounded by anxiety, and all of these factors combine to promote weight loss and general fatigue. Limb weakness, leading to difficulty manipulating food and raising it to the mouth, may make matters worse. Indeed, even in people without swallowing problems, limb weakness can cause weight loss because it reduces the efficiency of eating during mealtimes. Many of us 'graze' on snacks throughout the day. These subtle eating habits may well change because of impaired mobility, potentially causing a reduced calorie intake. At the time of diagnosis, we therefore advise people to cease any existing diets for weight restriction, as there are so many factors already promoting weight loss.

Can diet directly affect the course of MND?

There are many medical conditions such as heart disease, diabetes and stroke in which diet plays an important role in management and prevention. It is common sense that the food we take in, which is then metabolized to provide the essential building blocks for healthy tissues, could influence health and illness. The idea that nerve cells could be protected from injury by dietary modification is an inherently plausible one. Limited support for this idea comes from population studies showing that people whose diet contains higher levels of vitamins over many years are less likely to develop Alzheimer's disease. However, this is simply an association of one fact (high vitamin intake) with another (lower rates of dementia); it is not possible to conclude that there is a direct causal relationship. Neither is it evidence that certain diets are the 'cause' of neurodegenerative disease. High vitamin intake may simply be a marker for many other lifestyle or environmental factors such as not smoking or having a higher income. If diet is a factor in the development of neurodegenerative disease, it will be one part of a complex picture. Studies in which laboratory animals have been deprived of dietary antioxidants suggest that this leads to nerve damage. Antioxidants are chemicals which prevent damage to cells from dangerous 'free radicals' which are produced when cells are stressed or damaged. Despite the evidence suggesting that antioxidants could protect nerve cells from damage, trials in which vitamin E, carotene and other antioxidants have been used to treat neurodegenerative disease (including Parkinson's disease, Alzheimer's disease and MND) have all been a failure. This may be because the complexity of the cell death process in these diseases requires multiple pathways to be treated simultaneously or because it is simply too late to treat the process in this way once it has started. Therefore, there does not seem to be a way of directly affecting the process of nerve cell death in MND by dietary manipulation.

How can good nutritional care improve well-being for people living with MND?

Because there are no specific diets that will affect the course of MND, the advice offered to patients is aimed at maintaining good general health and well-being, and at preserving the important social function of mealtimes. First, it is critical not to adopt faddish diets suddenly which exclude core food groups. This may promote weight loss. At the time of diagnosis, when a minority of patients will have swallowing difficulties, there is no need for most people to change their diet. A consultation with a dietician may be helpful Because of the many different factors which act together to promote weight loss, the normal advice given by health care professionals to avoid high-fat foods can usually be modified for patients with MND. Extra treats, snacking and foods rich in carbohydrate and fats (e.g. chocolate puddings, cakes, and biscuits) are encouraged. There is no reason to give up alcohol, if it is drunk in moderation and continues to give pleasure and relaxation.

As MND progresses, the need to modify diet varies greatly depending on the individual pattern of muscle weakness. Difficulty using the hands to cut up and manipulate food will result in most people changing their food preference away from tougher meats such as steak. If mealtimes become daunting and cause fatigue, eating little and often can help. Having a snack between two smaller sized meals can avoid the need to struggle through a normal full-sized meal. Ensuring that an adequate amount of fluid is drunk is very important to aid good digestive function and prevent dehydration.

If the pattern of muscle weakness directly affects chewing and swallowing, a number of things can be done to make it easier. A combined approach involving advice from both a dietician and a SALT is valuable. They will provide individualized and step-by-step advice relevant to the particular stage of the illness. Initially, advice will include changing consistency of food away from dry flaky food such as crisps or dry bread which may catch at the back of the throat and trigger coughing. Eating small amounts at a time and concentrating on each mouthful, avoiding trying simultaneously to hold a conversation and adding extra moisture such as gravy or butter to food can all reduce the frequency of coughing episodes. Patients with neurological swallowing problems (there is no blockage to the passage of food but the co-ordination is defective) generally find liquids more difficult to cope with. Eating food which has a porridge-like consistency such as soft casseroles and stews or thick soups makes the process of swallowing easier. Similar textures can be achieved with mashed potato, and cooking vegetables and meat until tender and easy to cut.

Foods to avoid if there is significant swallowing difficulty

- Salads and raw vegetables, particularly lettuce

- Dry biscuits or crumbly bread

- Mixed textures, e.g. a thin soup with chunks of meat vegetables

- Hard food such as nuts or dry toast

- Stringy food that is difficult to chew, e.g. bacon rind or stringy beans

- Spicy food (may cause coughing)

Drinking water may become difficult. Interestingly, fizzy or icy drinks may be easier to swallow. Drinking smoothies or milk shakes is an excellent way to increase the consistency and ensure a good calorie intake. It is also possible to thicken everyday drinks such as tea and coffee, with a substance called Thick'n'Easy™. Once people have become accustomed to the strange sensation of drinking a thicker cup of coffee, it can be a useful way of preventing coughing while drinking.

If, despite these measures, a person with MND has started to find eating a chore and they are losing weight gradually, extra calories may be recommended. Adding extra calories to the normal diet is a good way to start, for example by mashing potatoes with cream instead of milk, or eating foods which contain natural fats, such as avocados. Supplements come in the form of drink cartons packed full of vitamins and calories. These are either milk based or fruity and can be drunk between meals or also taken as a soup.

What happens if people with MND are unable to take food by mouth?

If weakness of the muscles of speech and swallowing is significant, it can be impossible to prevent weight loss using the simple measures outlined above. A common solution to this problem for people living with MND is to consider direct delivery of food into the stomach using methods which bypass the swallowing mechanism. This is known as **enteral feeding**. The simplest way to do this is via a nasogastric tube (NG tube), a fine, soft tube which is placed up the nose and down into the stomach. It can be used as a short-term intervention. It may be offered to those too weak or frail to have a definitive procedure and where there is an urgent need to provide food and water to maintain comfort. However, it is not an ideal long-term solution as it can be uncomfortable, cause local irritation to the nose and palate and also frequently falls out and has to be replaced.

The most common technique used to support nutrition in people with MND goes by the highly technical term 'percutaneous endoscopic gastrostomy' (PEG), but is actually a very simple concept. An endoscope is an illuminated flexible fibre-optic cable attached to a camera. The endoscope is placed in the mouth, passed down the throat into the oesophagus and then into the stomach where the operator can see the indent made by a second person gently pressing down from the outside. When the correct position has been identified, under local anaesthetic, a small incision is made in the abdominal wall straight through into the stomach (hence 'percutaneously', or through the surface). A nylon thread is then passed through the incision. The endoscope then grasps the end in a pincer movement and is withdrawn slowly, still grasping the thread. Once the endoscope has been removed from the mouth there is a line of thread from the surface of the abdomen, through the incision hole, then running up through the stomach into the oesophagus and out of the mouth. A PEG tube is then attached to the thread at the mouth end. The other end of the thread is then pulled back gently but firmly. The PEG tube then threads its way back into the stomach and out of the incision hole to the surface of the abdomen. It is prevented from falling out by a small plastic disc inside the stomach. The thread is then removed from the PEG tube. A small plastic flange is slipped on to the PEG and is fastened close to the skin to keep the tube in place by preventing it from sliding back and forth (Fig. 4.2). A plastic cap is then attached to the loose end of the tube. 'Gastrostomy' literally means a hole or entry point into the stomach. The whole process takes no longer than approximately 20 minutes and is performed under sedation so that the patient will feel relaxed, but understand what is happening and be able to cooperate. It is usual to sleep for an hour or two afterwards and wake with no recollection of what has happened.

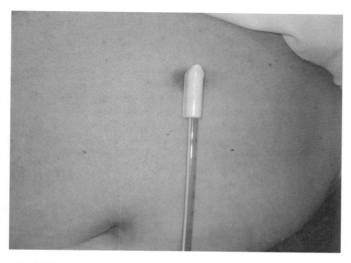

Figure 4.2 A PEG tube. A PEG tube sits comfortably under clothing and does not interfere with normal daily activity.

PEGs have been in wide use in medicine in the last 20 years in many different situations where swallowing is not possible, including in some people with stroke, cancer of the throat or oesophagus, oral surgery, and other neurological conditions such as multiple sclerosis. Extensive experience in specialist units has made PEG insertion a very safe procedure. However, in MND, timing of the procedure and patient selection are very important in making sure that a PEG has a real impact in maintaining well-being and is done with minimal risk of complications. Many studies have shown that the best outcomes are achieved when a PEG has been inserted at a fairly early stage, before it has become really necessary to rely on it. As with many other aspects of MND care, we emphasize planning ahead as being a better strategy than crisis management. At an earlier stage in the illness the person with MND will be able to lie flat more comfortably, breathing muscles will be stronger and the risk of complications such as a chest infection will be much lower. Generally, the risks of having a PEG are higher when the vital capacity, a measure of respiratory function (see below), is below 50 per cent of the predicted value. Therefore, we encourage people to make a choice before this stage has been reached. This means that many people may have a PEG inserted before they actually need to rely on it for most of their nutrition, and they can take a controlled approach to introducing nutritional supplements gradually through the PEG, while continuing to eat in the normal way. If the PEG is not being used, each day a small amount of water is flushed through the tube with a syringe to keep it clean.

Radiologically inserted gastrostomy (RIG) is a variant of the procedure which may be recommended if it has become difficult to lie flat because the breathing muscles have become weak. Prior to the RIG being inserted, a fine bore NG tube is placed through the nose and guided down to the stomach. This may feel slightly uncomfortable while it is being placed as it gives a strange sensation at the back of the throat, but once in position is not painful. The day before the RIG is inserted the patient is asked to drink a liquid which will show up on X-ray examination. If drinking is difficult it can be administered directly down the NG tube. On the next day, air is inserted into the stomach by way of the NG tube, inflating the stomach and moving it into the correct position. The skin of the abdomen is injected with local anaesthetic and a small incision is made in the skin through to the stomach. By using the X-ray as guidance, the gastrostomy tube is inserted directly into the stomach. The NG tube is then removed. Stitches called T-fasteners are then used to secure the stomach and tube. These are removed 10–14 days after the procedure. The RIG tube differs slightly from the PEG tube in the way it is secured. The RIG has a balloon type fixture which makes it easier to replace the tube if necessary without requiring another operation. Some people complain of abdominal pain which can radiate towards the shoulder blades. This is caused by the air in the stomach, but it soon disperses. There may also be a bit of tenderness from the stitches in the abdomen. The tube is then treated in exactly the same way as a PEG tube.

Many people with MND worry that an PEG or RIG tube might be difficult to manage without special medical training. However, the procedures involved in attaching feed to the PEG are very simple and can be learned by anybody. At the time of admission for PEG, the care team will provide the necessary training and liaise with colleagues based in the community (dieticians and District Nurses) who are available to support the continued use of the PEG even if disability progresses. Carers or family members can easily acquire the necessary skills to help the person with MND continue to use the PEG. All the necessary equipment will be provided and replaced by community teams.

Flushing the tube daily is important in order to keep the tube clean and free from blockage caused by food particles from the stomach. The water used for flushing the tube does not have to be sterile. It can be cool boiled water from the kettle. Once a week, to prevent the button from becoming ingrained into the lining of the stomach wall, the tube is rotated. For the first 7–10 days it is advisable to keep the site of the PEG or RIG as dry and clean as possible. After this time, once the wound has healed, it is then possible to have a bath or even go swimming as long as the wound site is thoroughly dried afterwards. A small 'key-hole' dressing may be applied to protect the area.

The dietician will work out the optimum amount of calories for each individual and recommend the best type of food depending on requirements for fibre and calories. There are various ways in which enteral feeding can be used. It is important that whichever plan is chosen fits the individual's lifestyle, which should not have to change dramatically. Even when eating and drinking is maintained and the PEG tube is only being flushed to keep it clear, it can be very useful in hot weather, when extra fluid will be needed. When enteral feeding is the mainstay of nutrition, the feed can be delivered at a set amount and at a regular speed by an electric pump, which can either be stationary or mounted on a portable stand or even in a back-pack. Depending on individual preference, feeding can occur through the night or during the day, either all at one time or split. Alternatively, a bag or bottle of feed can be hung from a stand and allowed to drip down the tube slowly under gravity without the need for an electric pump. Some people prefer 'bolus feeding', using a syringe to put larger amounts (50–100 ml at a time) through the tube, because it gives greater freedom and the feed can be given at meal times, helping to maintain normal social routines. The tube can also be used to administer medication. This is particularly useful if swallowing tablets has become difficult. Many types of tablets do come in liquid form and can be syringed into the tube. Remembering to flush the tube after the sticky medication is vital to prevent it from blocking.

The main aim of enteral feeding is to promote and maintain well-being rather than as a life-sustaining measure. However, it seems likely that people with MND who choose to have a PEG tube will be less susceptible to infection and generally less frail. In conjunction with other aspects of care, it is widely believed that having a PEG tube will extend life a little. If a PEG or RIG is inserted, it is possible to remove it if it is no longer wanted, following discussion and support to ensure that the implications of removing a tube are understood.

What are the factors in deciding whether to have enteral feeding?

Making any decision can be difficult, especially when an operation is involved. As with any aspect of decision making in MND, the starting point is to be well informed. An important point to keep in mind is that having a procedure leading to enteral feeding is a choice. Just because it *can* be done, it does not follow that it *should* be done in all cases. Even after extensive discussion with patients who we have felt were highly likely to benefit from a PEG placement, some people have decided that it is not for them. What has happened to these people? In general, they have continued to cope with MND in their own way without regretting their choice. This may have been despite a certain amount of avoidable weight loss and perhaps some extra difficulty with eating and drinking. It is impossible with any intervention to do more than speculate what would have happened had someone made a different decision. We can only base our advice on broad generalizations derived from large groups of patients. This has confirmed our view that for selected patients a PEG tube is a valuable way of maintaining well-being. While we give our advice in good faith, it is not always possible to be certain what is correct for individuals. That is why we always seek to support each person in their own choice, and our utmost concern is that whichever decision has been arrived at has been made with access to accurate information. It is also critical for the care team to know that the person with MND is fully in control of the decision themselves and that they are not acting in a certain way because they either are under pressure from family members or wish to please others.

We often find that people who are reluctant to consider a PEG tube have mistaken assumptions. For example, they think that managing the equipment is beyond them or that they will have to stop eating completely. Some people believe that tube feeding will prolong their life beyond a point when quality is maintained. Above all, the main reason for reluctance is a wish to postpone this difficult decision until later in the illness. Although we are very sympathetic to this wish, we know from experience that the best outcome is achieved if we support people in coming to an early decision.

 Nutrition in MND: key facts

- Swallowing is a complex manoeuvre, requiring a lot of muscles to be working in sequence. For some people living with MND this can become difficult

- Many people fear that they will choke to death. In our experience this does not happen

- People living with MND do lose weight for various reasons

- Eat small meals with snacks in between

- Change the consistency of food and fluids. Add supplements to diet

- Enteral feeding, through a fine tube called a PEG or RIG is a choice and depends on individual disease patterns and personal preferences

- The success of all these interventions requires careful timing

What sort of breathing difficulties can occur in MND?

The expansion of the chest cavity which occurs during normal breathing requires activation of the muscles of the chest wall and also the diaphragm (a large domed muscle which sits between the liver and the lungs). Any of these muscles can become affected in MND, leading to disturbances in breathing which can significantly affect well-being. For the majority of patients with MND it is this progressive loss of strength in respiratory muscles which is the chief factor in shortening their life. One of the earliest signs that breathing muscles may be affected by MND is disturbance in sleep. This may simply be that the person with MND wakes frequently through the night, which is termed **sleep fragmentation**. When we are awake, the rate, rhythm and depth of breathing is a combination of voluntary and involuntary muscle movement. The diaphragm is a largely involuntary muscle which functions to push down the liver into the abdomen so that the chest can expand. It is particularly important when we are lying flat such as during sleep, as without good diaphragmatic strength, the abdominal organs will limit the expansion of the chest. Diaphragmatic weakness leads to shallow breathing, with the result that the exchange of oxygen becomes inefficient. As well as leading to frequent waking, this results in a feeling of grogginess or lethargy on waking, early morning headaches, loss of appetite in the morning, frequently dropping off to sleep during the day and a general reduction in alertness. Someone with diaphragm weakness may be able to breathe normally when sitting upright during the day and unaware that they have a problem until they lie down flat. Occasionally, the first symptom of diaphragm weakness is a feeling of breathlessness on entering a swimming pool.

 Patient's perspective

Raymond is a 51-year-old lawyer who developed weakness and wasting of the left hand. This was very slowly progressive and it was about 2 years before the diagnosis of MND was confirmed when he developed a left foot drop and wasting of the right hand. Throughout this time he continued to work. In the third year of his illness, he mentioned that he had felt very uncomfortable on entering a swimming pool recently and that he was struggling to sing in his local choir. Even though his work seemed to be generally unaffected, he did admit that he needed an afternoon nap most days.

On examination, Raymond's vital capacity was normal sitting up. However, when he lay flat it dropped to 45 per cent of predicted, indicating that he was suffering from selective diaphragm weakness. Overnight sleep studies revealed that his oxygen levels dipped many times throughout the night. He was fitted with nocturnal non-invasive ventilation (NIV) with complete restoration of his sleep pattern and a greater feeling of mental vigour during the day. In retrospect, it was clear that his capacity for work had been progressively declining. With NIV, he was able to stay at work for a further 2 years, despite needing a wheelchair.

Breathlessness can occur for a number of reasons in MND, and is naturally a source of great anxiety for patients and their carers. Early on in MND, shortness of breath may arise at a time when we are not able to detect significant respiratory muscle weakness and may simply be due to an awareness by the patient that physical changes have occurred in the muscles of the chest. Given that breathing is normally an unconscious activity, this increased awareness can be quite intrusive and disturbing, and frequently leads to anxiety symptoms including panic attacks characterized by severe shortness of breath.

How are breathing symptoms assessed?

Clearly there are a number of potential reasons why someone with MND might suffer from poor sleep and, before deciding that it is due to breathing, it is important to consider other possibilities:

◆ Is it simply physical discomfort from difficulty in turning in bed? If we are unable to turn spontaneously this leads to arousal from sleep.

◆ Is there a significant disturbance of mood which is disturbing normal sleep? Patients with depression have difficulty getting off to sleep and also wake early in the morning. Some people with MND have experienced panic attacks which prevent them from sleeping. The quiet of the night time is frequently when we reflect on the day and take stock of our situation. Someone who is coping well with the diagnosis of MND during the day may find the night time suddenly produces a drop in their morale.

◆ The physical changes associated with MND often lead to a reduction in physical activity and a change in the normal rhythm of life, which may be enough to explain a change in someone's sleeping pattern.

To aid us in deciding who may be suffering from sleep fragmentation due to weakness of breathing muscles, we measure **vital capacity (VC)** with a test in which a piece of equipment called a spirometer is used to measure how much air can be expelled by the lungs in one breath. Measurement of VC should always be taken in the context of what is normal for height, race, age and gender. Therefore, we usually express it as a percentage of predicted, rather than as an absolute numerical value. It is important to realize that the VC will decline progressively in the majority of patients as MND progresses. However, the extent to which this decline in VC is associated with actual respiratory symptoms is highly variable and not always easy to predict in individual patients. Many patients progress through their illness without experiencing any specific symptoms relating to breathing despite low VC levels. This probably reflects variation in how we adapt to respiratory changes, but also the balance between diaphragmatic and other muscle weakness. A variety of other tests may be carried out either in an MND clinic or by specialist chest physicians, depending on the facilities available. In addition, we use a simple questionnaire to detect those patients with MND who may have early breathing muscle weakness (see box).

Simple sleep and breathing questionnaire

1. Are you breathless (a) at rest, (b) on minimal exertion, (c) under moderate exertion?

2. Are you breathless when lying flat?

3. Do you sleep well at night? If not why not?

4. Do wake refreshed in the morning?

5. Do you drop off to sleep frequently during the day, e.g. while a passenger in a car, watching TV, reading?

How are breathing symptoms managed?

As with all other aspects of the management of MND, the starting point is explanation. It is important for people to see their own disease in the context of the clinical variability of MND as a whole. This means appreciating that some people with MND do not experience significant respiratory difficulties at all, and that for many people symptomatic control of breathing only needs to be addressed at the very end of life. It also means understanding that interventions such as assisted ventilation are a choice, and it is for the doctor and patient to work in partnership to agree what is appropriate.

The management of sleep fragmentation due to breathing muscle weakness has been greatly improved by the use of **non-invasive ventilation (NIV)**. At the simplest level, this consists of delivering air to the chest at a higher

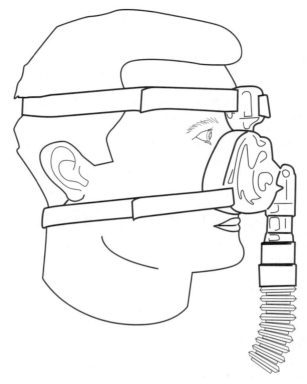

Figure 4.3 Non-invasive ventilation. A nasal mask delivers air at pressure to help ease the work of breathing and restore good ventilation to the lungs.

pressure than that normally achieved during breathing. This is done by fitting a tightly sealed mask over the nose (Fig. 4.3). The aim is gently to force the chest to expand, taking over some of the work of breathing and restoring good oxygen delivery. The selection of patients who will benefit from NIV is a skilled task best performed by a respiratory physician in partnership with an MND specialist. As with any other treatment for the symptoms of MND, having NIV is a choice that has to be carefully considered within the context of the illness as a whole. Some patients simply do not like the feeling of having their chest passively expanded by high pressure and do not tolerate the equipment (which is also quite noisy and can certainly disrupt the sleep pattern of bed partners!). The aim of NIV is to restore sleep patterns, reduce daytime somnolence and generally improve well-being. The incidence of chest infections is also likely to be lower if NIV is used. It is likely that NIV can improve the length of survival for patients with MND, but this is still being tested in clinical studies. The main aim of offering NIV at present is not to prolong life but to improve symptoms.

As indicated above, shortness of breath can have a number of origins in MND. Reassurance that an increased awareness of the breathing muscles is not in itself a sign of impending respiratory failure is an important part of the management of breathing difficulties. If anxiety is a significant component, then it is sometimes appropriate for drug treatments aimed at anxiety management to be used. Beta-blockers blunt the 'adrenaline response' (which promotes an increase in pulse and breathing rate in response to fright and fear) and can prevent anxiety progressing to a full-blown panic attack. Benzodiazepines (Valium and related drugs) have a general effect in reducing anxiety levels and promoting sleep, though they should be used cautiously if breathing muscle weakness is present. In the management of the terminal phase of MND, morphine is an excellent drug for relieving breathing-related symptoms. However, like benzodiazepines, it can suppress breathing function, and doctors, nurses, people with MND and their carers will have to consider the pros and cons of using such drugs, with symptom control being the priority.

 Patient's perspective

Jamie is a 24-year-old man who has developed MND at an unusually young age. He has a wife and a small baby, and 9 months after the diagnosis of MND has had to give up work as a mechanic because his arms are weak. He has great difficulty coming to terms with the illness and has appeared very frightened during clinic visits. Our attempts to explore his fears have not so far resulted in him being able to talk openly about the effect of MND on his life. He prefers to 'take one day at time' and not think about the future. He was seen in clinic earlier than planned because on two occasions in 1 week he had been admitted to his local hospital with severe shortness of breath in the night. On each occasion he had been allowed home the next day.

In clinic we measured his vital capacity, which was normal. We showed Jamie the charts on which we had documented that his breathing muscles had remained strong despite his arms growing progressively weaker. We explored his fears. During the quiet hours of the night, Jamie would begin to think about the effect of MND on shortening his life. He would become more aware of his breathing, which would become more rapid until he was fighting for his breath and was convinced that he was suddenly going to die.

We explained to Jamie that patients with MND do not suddenly stop breathing and that he currently showed no signs of breathing muscle weakness. We helped Jamie draw up an advance directive in which he expressed his wish to have every treatment possible to keep him well, except that, as with the majority of patients with MND, he did not ever wish to be incapacitated by having a tracheostomy and permanent ventilation. His panic attacks disappeared and subsequent clinic visits have been more relaxed. Jamie has been much more confident in openly discussing his fears.

Breathing: summary points

- Not all patients with MND experience symptoms due to weak breathing muscles

- At various points in the illness it is common to experience anxiety about breathing, which can even lead to panic attacks

- All patients with MND should have access to expert support from a respiratory team working in partnership with an MND specialist clinic

- Selected patients benefit from non-invasive ventilation as a symptom control measure. Its effect in prolonging life is still under assessment

How can excess secretions be relieved?

We produce several litres of saliva per day, and most of this is swallowed without any further thought. While many MND patients do not experience excess secretions, in some people with MND, the reflex swallowing mechanism may be impaired. This can lead to discomfort when saliva pools at the back of the throat, and the only way to clear this may be to allow it to come out through the mouth into a tissue. If this saliva is not replaced by taking in more fluid, dehydration can sometimes result, especially during hot weather. It is also a major source of social embarrassment.

There are a number of ways to manage excess saliva, but none of these are perfect and it can be a difficult area of management. The first principle is to decide if the problem is one of excess thick secretions or of excess thin secretions. Thick secretions can be made less troublesome by avoiding dehydration by remembering to drink plenty of fluids, by sucking on boiled sweets and also by avoiding dairy products. Pineapple juice contains an enzyme which can break down thick saliva. Steam inhalations can also help keep the mouth and throat moist. Excess thin secretions can be treated with a variety of drugs, but the side effects (not least that of a dry mouth) can be troublesome. Hyoscine, which can be prescribed as skin patches or tablets, is contained in 'sea-sickness' pills, and dry mouth is a side effect which can be usefully employed in patients with excess saliva. Unfortunately, many patients, especially the elderly, feel quite drowsy at the doses required to have good effect. Atropine is a drug with a similar effect. It is used a eye drops for the treatment of glaucoma and these drops can be put under the tongue to provide rapid but short-term relief of salivation. This use of atropine should only be tried under medical advice. Amitriptiline is an antidepressant which also has the side effect of drying the mouth and can be a useful treatment, especially in those who cannot sleep at night. If neither of these work, glycopyrrolate can be tried, but this must be given by injection. Lastly, botulinum toxin can be injected into the salivary gland to shut off saliva production. As well as being quite a drastic solution, this requires an injection from a specialist and may not be widely available.

The altered feeling that arises in the back of the throat due to muscle weakness and stiffness and the pooling of saliva can make people feel very uneasy, and it is common to worry that sudden choking will lead to a complete loss of the ability to breathe. While occasionally very frightening choking episodes do occur in selected patients with stiff throat muscles which can go into spasm, this does not result in a sudden loss of breathing or sudden death. It is very important to appreciate that this feeling of throat spasm will spontaneously resolve, usually within a minute. Conscious attempts to relax and making swallowing motions can help bring an episode to an end. The minority of patients who have frequent and troublesome throat spasms are sometimes prescribed lorazepam (one of the benzodiazepine family of drugs) which can be administered under the tongue for rapid effect.

What is the best treatment for cramps and fasciculations?

Fasciculations are irregular and chaotic twitching of muscle fibres. Because muscle is an 'excitable' tissue (that means that electrical impulses can be transmitted to muscle as part of its normal function) it is quite normal for muscle to twitch occasionally. Exercise, caffeine, alcohol, various medications and temperature changes can all increase the probability that muscle will twitch. The degree to which muscle will twitch in this way seems to vary between individuals. As mentioned in Chapter 1, excessive twitching of muscle occurs in the syndrome known as **benign fasciculations**. However, in the context of wasting and weakness, fasciculations are an important feature of the diagnosis of MND. The degree to which people with MND are aware of fasciculation is very variable, with many patients remaining unaware until their attention is drawn to muscle twitching by doctors. However, for some people, fasciculations can be highly intrusive. In the first instance, it is important for people to appreciate that fasciculations can worsen because of anxiety as well as all of the things mentioned above. There is no clear relationship between the intensity of fasciculations as experienced by the patient and the degree of motor neuron damage. As the disease progresses, it is usual for fasciculations to recede into the background. Most people are reassured by this knowledge and do not require specific treatment. However, a few people are sufficiently disturbed by fasciculations that they require drugs to suppress them. Beta-blockers can be effective, as can the drug baclofen (see below).

Spasticity is the term used for muscles which have increased resistance to passive movement. This means that when the leg or arm is stretched out it tends to stiffen up. This can lead to difficulty in dressing and also instability. People with stiff legs are at risk of falling because they cannot adjust their centre of gravity in response to the need to change position or direction, and tend to move their body above the waist while their legs are rooted to the ground, with obvious results.

Cramps are sudden tightening feelings in individual muscles which can be very painful and leave the muscle bruised and sore. They are usually activated by movement and changes in posture which involve stretching. Cramps are particularly troublesome at night in bed. As with fasciculations, cramps are often most prominent early in the disease and frequently fade into the background, except in those patients with upper motor neuron predominant disease such as PLS, in which case they can be an ongoing problem. Spasticity and cramps are related phenomena that are caused by a loss of motor control from the brain to the spinal cord. The treatments are therefore similar. Both are made worse by cold weather, anxiety or frustration, caffeine and certain medical drugs (such as inhalers for asthma). Physiotherapy has a role to play because keeping a limb mobile and supple and extending it through its full range of motion regularly, while it may provoke cramps during the therapy session, tends to make them less likely at other times. Tendons are fibrous tissue which attaches the body of a muscle to its point of insertion in a joint or bone. Immobility leads to tendon shortening and raises the tension in muscles during movement, making cramps and spasticity more likely. In addition to physiotherapy and simple measures such as preventing limbs getting cold and minimizing caffeine intake, some drugs can help. It should be emphasized that for most people with MND cramps are a short-lived problem and tend to fade. Reassurance and explanation are usually all that is required. However, **baclofen** is a drug which can be useful, though it does have side effects. It works by promoting the activity of an inhibitory neurotransmitter called GABA. Since this is present throughout the nervous system, raising its level leads to drowsiness. This often wears off, but many people find it difficult to cope with. Baclofen must be given in low doses initially and then increased very slowly under the supervision of a neurologist. In special circumstances, baclofen can be delivered directly to the spinal cord using an implantable pump device. This is a specialist treatment which is only suitable for patients who are not walking and who have a slowly progressive or static neurological condition. There are a range of other drugs that can be tried, including tizanidine, gabapentin, phenytoin and dantrolene. **Botulinum toxin** works by paralysing the muscles that are overactive. This can be very helpful in relieving spasticity but, since it further weakens motor function, it is usually only suitable for people who have lost the ability to walk.

Does MND cause pain?

The degeneration of motor nerves in MND is not in itself a painful process. Any pain and discomfort that occurs in MND is therefore a secondary consequence of weakness and poor mobility, and is therefore in principle completely manageable. The most common source of pain and discomfort experienced by MND patients arises in weight-bearing joints, particularly the shoulder, back and hip. The shoulder joint is like a ball in a shallow cup and is buttressed and stabilized by strong muscles which enfold it. If there is weakness and wasting in any of the muscles around the shoulder, this can lead to joint instability, irritation and inflammation of the joint surface, and consequently pain. Many patients with MND never experience joint pain and those that do often find that it is associated with a particular phase of the illness and tends to fade into the background with time. Musculoskeletal or mechanical pain such as this is best managed using a combination of exercises to mobilize the joint and simple analgesia such as paracetamol, and anti-inflammatory drugs such as ibuprofen. As with any pain management, the best approach is to treat the pain when it is at a low level. Once pain has built up, it is always more difficult to control, and stronger drugs are required with more side effects. Many patients find that regular paracetamol (two tablets every 6 hours) is a safe and effective way of controlling pain.

Another source of mechanical pain is tendon shortening. This occurs most commonly in the shoulder, ankle and the hand. If a group of muscles around a joint is weak, the range of movement around that joint will decrease and tendons will begin to shorten. This is experienced as a feeling of tightness. If the joint is moved outside of the range of voluntary action, for example the shoulder during dressing, this stretches the already tight tendon and causes pain. The best way to manage this problem is by early identification of those patients who are most at risk, introduction of passive exercise which can be taught to carers by a physiotherapist, and the simple pain relief medications mentioned above.

Particular problems with mechanical pain and discomfort arise at night. The average person turns in their sleep every 30 minutes or so. Even early in the disease when mobility during the day may be good, sleep can be disrupted by discomfort arising from not being able to turn efficiently. This is one of the contributing factors to sleep fragmentation.

Does MND lead to mood disturbance?

Being diagnosed with MND and the experience of coping with physical decline can reasonably be described as a major 'life event'. It is appropriate for people with MND to feel the range of emotions that one would normally associate with a major bereavement such as the loss of a close relative. In this case, the sense of bereavement will be about the loss of future aspirations. Anger ('it's not fair'), questioning ('why me?'), guilt ('have I brought this on myself?') and frustration are all normal and expected emotions at this time (see Chapter 3). Periods of tearfulness are common and may be highly appropriate. However, it is common when people become ill from any cause (heart attacks, diabetes, multiple sclerosis, etc.) that there is a greater risk of appropriate mood disturbance turning into significant depression. Given that this is a treatable problem, it is very important to identify those patients with MND who may benefit from treatment. Some neurologists and many GPs will be experienced in the management of depression but, where there is doubt, the advice of a psychiatrist may be helpful. Some clinics have a clinical psychologist as part of the multidisciplinary team.

How can doctors distinguish between normal sadness and depression?

Some people seem predisposed to developing depression. Like many things it is probably a mixture of genetic make-up and external experience. People who have had a major depressive illness in the past (e.g. depression following childbirth) are more likely to suffer one again. Just like other illnesses, depression sometimes just seems to arise out of nowhere. This is referred to by psychiatrists as 'endogenous' depression. A severe and disabling mood disturbance in response to life events is called 'reactive' depression. It is not easy, nor especially relevant in the context of MND, to make the distinction between the two types of depression, but it is vital to identify significant mood disturbance that will respond to treatment. The key symptoms that help identify treatable mood disturbance are tearfulness, sleep disturbance, loss of motivation, inability to enjoy things and weight loss. It will be obvious that many of these problems occur in MND for other reasons. Thus a trial of treatment may be the only way of distinguishing true depressive symptoms from an adjustment reaction.

What is the role of palliative care services in symptom control?

Palliative care teams are run by doctors and nurses with special training in symptom control and end of life issues. They are often based in hospices, but parallel teams are often found in larger hospitals. Depending on the way that local practice has evolved, the level of involvement of palliative care teams in managing MND can vary considerably. Some of the most renowned experts in the field of MND management worldwide are palliative care specialists, while other hospice teams will only have very sporadic experience of neurological conditions. For people living with MND, the involvement of palliative care teams sometimes raises unnecessary fears. It should not mean that neurological care will cease, nor does it necessarily indicate that the illness is in the terminal phase. Much of the work of palliative care medicine is in supporting people in their homes. Treatable symptoms in MND can arise at any stage of the illness, and experts in symptom control should therefore be available to people with MND at the most appropriate time for the individual. Furthermore, a range of services are available through palliative care which are not found in other settings, including massage, individual counselling and respite for carers.

However, MND can be a challenge to palliative care teams who are more used to looking after patients with cancer. This may simply be because of unfamiliarity with the disease. MND also poses a challenge because predicting the time at which people are likely to die is very inexact, and hospices, which have scarce resources, generally only offer care to people within a defined period at the end of their life. There is a sense in which MND is a terminal illness for a much longer period than many cancers, which often have a phase of treatment and remission before recurrence leads to the terminal phase. Another challenge for palliative care teams is that increasing numbers of patients with MND are being treated with relatively invasive strategies such as NIV and PEG.

In this chapter, we have looked at drugs and other specific medical treatments that can alleviate the symptoms of MND. In the next chapter we look at how the multidisciplinary team can help people with MND maintain their independence.

5

Maintaining well-being

Introduction

The effects on quality of life of a debilitating and complex disease such as MND vary greatly from one individual to another. Clearly one factor is the pattern of progression and pace of change of the disease itself. Another important factor is variation in individual personality, and we all respond to adversity with different degrees of resilience. Our ability to control these two aspects of the disease is limited. However, access to the wide range of skills in the multidisciplinary care team can be a major determinant of well-being for people living with MND.

Can exercise help maintain muscle strength?

Our everyday experience tells us that physical fitness makes a difference to how we feel and to our health. Body builders and athletes train to enhance muscle performance, and physiotherapists help people back on their feet after joint replacement operations, using controlled exercise programmes to strengthen muscles that have not been working. Is it therefore possible that repetitively driving muscles made weak by MND could strengthen these muscles or prevent them from getting worse? The reason that muscles become weak and wasted in MND is that the nerve normally connecting the muscle to the spinal cord has become disconnected. Unfortunately, this means that no amount of stimulation of the muscle itself will make a difference as the muscle cannot work without this connection to the nervous system. It is sometimes claimed that electrical stimulation of the muscle using various pieces of equipment such as 'faradic stimulators' will help re-establish nerve muscle connection. However, in MND, there is no evidence that this is of any benefit.

Could exercise be harmful?

As mentioned in Chapter 2, the most prevalent theory about the cause of MND is that individuals who get the disease carry a genetic profile which makes them susceptible. Though it is far from clear at present, some researchers have found evidence that athletic people may be more susceptible than people who lead a more sedentary lifestyle. Even if true, this is likely to be quite a weak effect, but it might indicate that genetic profiles which promote athletic prowess in youth, for example by allowing muscle to be efficient in the use of energy, may be harmful later in life. Because of this, some people worry that exercising muscles affected by nerve degeneration through MND could accelerate the disease process. There is not a shred of evidence to support this, however. In the limited number of studies in which programmed exercise has been tried in patients it did not obviously lead to more rapid progression. In studies in which SOD1 mutant mice were allowed to spend all day on a treadmill this actually seemed to improve survival a little! We have certainly had a few very enthusiastic patients who have exercised extremely vigorously, and they have not come to harm through this, though neither have they obviously benefited.

What sort of exercise is likely to be helpful?

Whatever will eventually be concluded about whether athleticism is part of the complex risk profile for MND, it is clear that exercise does not have an obvious effect on disease progression. However, there are clear reasons why remaining as fit as possible is a good idea. Exercise enhances general well-being, promotes a healthy sleep pattern and stimulates the appetite. Therefore, while we do not suggest that people suddenly take up new forms of exercise, we do encourage people newly diagnosed with MND to continue their normal exercise programme, perhaps to make it more regular. Swimming is a particularly beneficial form of exercise because many muscles are used simultaneously and because being in the water can overcome the mechanical disadvantage of lifting heavy muscles (a minor form of weightlessness that astronauts experience in space) and allow a much fuller range of movements. Even if swimming is not possible, walking in a shallow pool with assistance or sitting in a shallow warm pool and moving the limbs through a wide arc can be very beneficial. Clearly, swimming pools with their slippery floors can be very hazardous places for anyone with difficulty walking, and extreme caution and a willingness to have a helper are very important. Other forms of exercise which are worth considering include an exercise bicycle. Although the effects of exercise will mostly be non-specific in promoting general well-being, people with MND who have a lot of stiffness and cramps should find that controlled exercise will improve these symptoms to some extent.

How will MND affect my sexual relationship?

Sexuality is a subject that we all find difficult. Nurses and doctors are notoriously bad at broaching the subject with their patients and assume that if there is a problem the patient will bring it up. Health care professionals may feel that they do not have the relevant expertise to talk about sex. Natural discomfort with the subject may also arise from an unwillingness to draw upon knowledge from a personal perspective. Yet many studies have shown that patients want to talk about sex but do not know how to discuss it either. This lack of communication can only lead to frustration.

Many of us have been in a relationship when the intimate side has been difficult and less pleasurable than expected due to anxiety, pain, excess alcohol, tiredness, or any number of other reasons. Whatever the cause, it will certainly have an effect on how we feel and behave the following day. If the problem is a recurrent one, it can lead to one or both of the partners feeling worried and insecure about their whole relationship, not just about the sexual aspect. On the other hand, if things are going well, we tend to take a good sex life for granted. A diagnosis of MND affects people in profound ways and means dealing not only with physical loss but possibly also loss of identity. Roles within the family may have to change. There may be a change in status as the breadwinner or career person, and periods of grieving for the loss of the physical ability to work. Adjusting to this may be challenging, especially if the physical changes of MND occur at a rapid rate.

In the clinic we often become aware of the strain that MND imposes on relationships. We try to encourage people to talk about their worries and anxieties with their partner. No one should have to cope with problems on their own. Talking about intimate and very personal issues can make both partners in a relationship feel very vulnerable. A sense of humour can be very useful when talking about sexual problems, and avoiding a critical and negative tone and concentrating on the positive things makes things easier. Phrases such as 'It really feels lovely when you do that' or 'Next time can we try it like this' are examples. MND does not affect a person's sexual function in the physical sense. Feeling and sensation remain the same. It is still possible to achieve an erection and orgasm. Depending on strength and stamina, what may change is the technique of lovemaking. It may be necessary to change from familiar positions. As the disease progresses, it might be less comfortable to have intercourse in bed; an easy-chair or sofa can be more supportive. Many people have talked about the fact that due to their limited movement is has been more difficult to achieve a climax. Penetration is not always necessary for sexual fulfilment; the use of a vibrator or stimulator can help achieve an orgasm with less energy expenditure. In addition, masturbation can be a natural way to explore your own body and understand the kind of touch which gives pleasure and relaxation. The message is, do not be afraid to try something new.

We have sex for many different reasons; to express love, to relax, to show we care and are attracted to someone, to reproduce, and to give and receive satisfaction. Apart from reproduction, all these can be achieved without having sex. There may be times when sex is just too stressful to be pleasurable. Even if you decide to give it a break just to take the pressure off, don't give up on flirting, flattery or sexy comments to your partner. Keeps things ticking over until you both feel like starting again.

Much of this discussion has been focused on a partnership. However, there are many people who are not in a relationship and are able to give themselves pleasure by masturbating using fantasies, sexy magazines, films and vibrators. This is an essential way to relieve tension. In some situations, this can become difficult due to weakness of the hands or arms. This situation can lead to great frustration. Visiting a sex worker is an option that some people choose, particularly when deprived of human contact and sexually frustrated. It is not illegal, but it is advisable to avoid red light districts or street workers where crime is rife. All usual precautions, such as wearing a condom for men, are essential to avoid a sexually transmitted disease (STD).

 Sexual relationships and MND: key facts

- MND does not affect sexual function

- It may be necessary to change the technique to enable you to fulfil your relationship

- Think of different positions to make intimacy more comfortable

- It is really important to talk; talk to your partner and/or whoever you feel at ease with

- When talking about your relationship with your partner emphasize the positive aspects

- Seek guidance from a health professional if unsure or anxious

Is continence affected by MND?

Having been given the diagnosis of MND, many people are comforted at least by the fact that they will remain continent. This seems to be a crucial element to maintaining dignity and self-respect. People with MND continue to have 'normal' sensations and awareness of the need to empty their bladder and have their bowels open. The problems encountered are more of a practical kind to do with mobility. For these problems there are many practical solutions that can make going to the toilet a little easier. Hand rails can be fitted in strategic positions to provide extra stability and support in lowering and standing up in the toilet and bathroom. These rails are also useful for support when negotiating steps. A community occupational therapist (OT) often supplies this equipment, which can also be purchased from specialist chemists. Raised toilet seats, which fit on top of the original seat, reduce the distance needed to lower oneself and can also make standing up easier as there is less strain on the legs. These do not require special fitting and can be removed easily. A commode resembles a chair on wheels with a hole in the seat and has arms on either side and a seat back. Using a commode can increase the feeling of security by giving extra support while sitting over the toilet. Sometimes people use a commode as a way to access the lavatory, or keep it close to the bed, making going to the lavatory at night much safer. Having a commode should not compromise privacy. If the arms are weak or the hand grip is poor, simple things that we take for granted such as wiping our bottom can become very difficult. Getting help from others can cause a great deal of distress and embarrassment. A Closimat Toilet washes and dries the bottom after elimination by sending a spray of warm water from under the rim of the toilet bowl. Once the bottom is washed, it then sends a stream of hot air which dries it, leaving the bottom feeling fresh and clean! Though costly, people often feel that it is worth every penny as it enables them to maintain their privacy, independence and dignity. Urinals can be very useful and reduce the need to transfer onto the toilet or commode. For men this is very easy as a plastic urinal is convenient and can be used with ease. Alternatively an improvised ordinary bottle of fabric conditioner, which usually has a handle on the side, could be used. It is a little known fact that there are about 20 different types of female urinal. As you can imagine, these are different from the male urinal but can be equally easy to use provided the correct size and shape is acquired. If sitting in a wheelchair, wearing a skirt makes the use of the urinal possible. It is also helpful to purchase pants with a flap down the front. Information about where these can be purchased is available from the District Nurse or Continence Advisor. A slipper bed pan is used by ladies while in bed. Using any of the female urinals is 'an art' and can take some time to master. Don't give up. If worried about spillage, place an 'inco' sheet or plastic bag underneath to catch any dribbles. The District Nurse can provide sachets which look like a tea bag and, when placed in the bottom of the urinal, changes the urine to a gel-like consistency. If there is arm or hand weakness it is sometimes more convenient for men to wear a sheath, which resembles a condom with a hole at the end. This is fixed to a bag attached to the leg, discretely positioned inside the trouser. Sheaths are quite easy to apply and can be helpful when going out or travelling, as it is not necessary to rely on assistance from a partner or carer. The key to success when using a 'uri' sheath is to ensure that you have the correct size. All makes vary slightly, but to ensure that it will not leak take one minute to hold the sheath and penis. The warmth of the hand ensures the glue softens slightly and becomes secure.

If there is an event or occasion which you are really looking forward to, but anxious about the practicalities of using the toilet, there is a solution. Desmopressin, a drug which comes in the form of a nasal spray, is similar to a hormone found naturally in the body and works by decreasing the production of urine in the kidneys. Desmopressin has to be used with caution and as an occasional short-term measure only. It can also be taken before bedtime to enable people to sleep through the night without having to get up to pass urine. It is wise to talk to your GP about taking this drug as there are contraindications, such as high blood pressure or heart disease. The amount of fluids taken in may have to be limited.

A catheter is a soft plastic or rubber tube that is inserted into the urethra and up into the bladder to drain the urine. Urinary catheters are sometimes recommended as a way to manage urinary incontinence and urinary retention in both men and women. However, catheters are generally not the first choice for continence management in MND for several reasons. Control and sensation are normal and therefore it should be possible to maintain good continence using the methods already referred to. Urinary catheters carry a significant risk of infection and are therefore best avoided. Additionally, although having a catheter does not make intercourse impossible, it may make an already strained situation that bit more tense. For women, the catheter tube can be taped back out of the way, for men it can be bent back along the shaft of the penis and secured in place by using a condom. If catheterization is the preferred method of choice and it is to be used over a long period of time, a suprapubic catheter may be an appropriate solution. This is basically an indwelling catheter that is placed directly into the bladder through the skin of the abdomen. The catheter is inserted above the pubic bone into the bladder. This type of catheter must be placed by a surgeon and involves a small procedure under local anaesthetic. There is evidence to suggest that there is a reduced risk of acquiring a urinary tract infection with a suprapubic catheter because the tube is not in direct contact with the genital area. Needless to say, cleanliness is an essential part of the management for either type of

Table 5.1 'Adequate' daily intake of fluids

Weight		Fluid intake			
Stones	kg	ml	Fluid oz.	Pints	Mugs
6	38	1190	42	2.1	4
7	45	1275	49	2.5	5
8	51	1446	56	2.75	5–6
9	57	1786	63	3.1	6
10	64	1981	70	3.5	7
11	70	2179	77	3.75	7–8
12	76	2377	84	4.2	8
13	83	2575	91	4.5	9
14	89	2773	98	4.9	10

Adapted from Abrams P and Klevmar B (1996). Frequency volume charts: an indispensable part of lower urinary tract assessment. *Scandinavian Journal of Neurology* **179**:47–53.

catheter. The tube and surrounding area must be cleansed daily with soapy water, rinsed and dried thoroughly. The suprapubic catheter can be covered with a dry gauze cut half way in and placed around the tube in a so-called key-hole dressing. The skin around the catheter must be regularly inspected for signs of infection. It often has a 'crusty layer' to it, but this is normal. If it looks red and sore and feels warm to the touch, a localized infection is possible and the District Nurse should be informed. It is vitally important to drink adequate fluid. Table 5.1 gives some guideline for an 'adequate' daily intake and, for someone of average build, is accurate to within 10 per cent. Very overweight people may need special advice, and individual levels of activity should be taken into account. Hot weather can dramatically increase the need for fluid. During a hot summers day, we may lose 1–2 litres through perspiration.

How can constipation be prevented?

Constipation is a common complaint for people living with MND and it arises through multiple mechanisms. Understanding how the bowel works can really help in the management and prevention of constipation. The large intestine has two main functions: excretion of waste products and recovery of water and electrolytes. By the time ingested food has reached the large intestine, roughly 90 per cent of its water has been absorbed, but a considerable amount of water and electrolytes such as sodium remain and must be recovered by absorption by the large intestine.

Formation and storage of faeces

The ingested food is moved through the large intestine, by a process called peristalsis in which the muscle of the bowel wall contracts and relaxes in a co-ordinated way so that food residue is pushed along. There is a direct link between the length of time the faeces are in the large intestine and the amount of water that is absorbed. For example, spicy food containing chillies stimulates the bowel, increasing peristalsis and food transit and resulting in less water being absorbed and a softer product. Diarrhoea is an extreme case of this problem. Likewise, if the faeces remain in the bowel for a longer time, more water is absorbed and the faeces become dehydrated, smaller and harder, in extreme cases resembling 'rabbit droppings!'. An ideal type of stool is somewhere in between: well formed and 'sausage' like. We all have our individual routines or bowel 'habit'. What is considered normal for one person may be a problem for another. A reasonable definition of the range of normal bowel action is 'no more than 3 times a day or no less than 3 times a week'. There are several reasons why people with MND become constipated.

- Reduced intake of fluids. If the skin on the back of the hand is gently pinched and stays in the pinched position for a second or two once released, it is a sign that more fluid needs to be drunk. Urine ought to be a light straw colour. Dark urine is another indication of dehydration.

- Change in diet. 'Western' diets are much lower in fibre than is ideal. Fatigue or difficulty in swallowing may lead to a reduction in fibre intake. Breakfast cereals such as Weetabix™, softened with milk, and bananas are a good way to increase the dietary fibre in the diet. A dietitian can provide advice.

- Reduced activity levels can have a significant effect on bowel action because peristalsis is aided by the body's natural motion. Gentle bowel massage can help to maintain bowel routine. This technique was apparently invented by W. K. Kellogg who was said to carry out regular bowel massages using a cannon ball rolled around his abdomen! A more practical method is to use the heel of the palm of the hand and gently massage in a clockwise direction (the same direction of the bowel and waves of peristalsis). Rocking back and forth in a chair may have the same effect.

- Certain medications, such as the painkiller codeine (and similar drugs of the morphine family), can cause constipation by a direct pharmacological effect on the bowel. If such medicines are absolutely necessary for comfort, increased fluid and dietary fibre or even a laxative may be required. Paracetamol and anti-inflammatory drugs such as ibuprofen do not cause constipation.

- Psychological factors. It is common experience that anxiety can increase bowel activity, but one's state of mind can also have a negative effect on bowel function. Furthermore, if getting to the lavatory is more of a practical challenge than it once was, there is a tendency to ignore the urge to open the bowels. If regular bowel habits are broken, this can have a significant effect in slowing bowel activity.

- Nerves which are part of the autonomic (unconscious) nervous system drive the contraction of bowel muscle. It is a theoretical possibility that these nerves could be damaged in MND, though this seems to be unusual.

Each person has their own bowel routine reflecting their individual lifestyle. Any change in routine, even holidays or a change in job, can require a period of physical readjustment. Re-establishing a routine can take time. The very best time to have your bowels opened is in the morning, 20–30 minutes after breakfast or a hot drink. This is when the waves of peristalsis are at their strongest due to the 'gastro-colic reflex' in which food received into the stomach promotes a direct message to the large bowel to contract, stimulating the whole length of the digestive tract into action after a nights rest. Attempting a bowel action at night, when the bowels are at their most sluggish, is less likely to be successful. Laxatives can aid in establishing a routine but must be taken with caution. For example, a laxative may be taken before bed with the expectation of a result the next morning. When this does not occur, more laxatives are taken in the morning and subsequently, until a soft and 'explosive' result is finally achieved, typically a couple of days later. All laxatives take between 12 and 36 hours to work, so patience is advised. It is also important to choose the correct type of laxative, as there are several different mechanisms of action. Stimulant laxatives work directly on the large intestine to strengthen the waves of contraction and reduce the length of time faeces are in the bowel, and thus the amount of water reabsorbed. Bulk-forming laxatives are fibre based and enable faeces to pass through the bowel more easily by giving the bowel something to contract against. They also act as a medium for the growth of bacteria in the gut, which adds to the overall mass of the stool. Faecal softeners allow fat and fluids to penetrate the stool, lowering the surface tension of the stool, making it soft, bulky and easier to pass. Osmotic laxatives reduce the amount of water which is absorbed into the large intestine, thus keeping the stool more hydrated and hence softer. District Nurses are trained to choose the best laxative depending on the cause of constipation. A common problem for people living with MND is difficulty in generating muscle force in the pelvis to push down and expel the faeces, in which cases a stimulant laxative can be effective. Enemas and suppositories are sometimes used if constipation has not been relieved by simple methods. An enema is a small amount of liquid inserted directly into the rectum which both stimulates and lubricates the bowel, enabling the faeces to be passed with ease. Although this sounds easy enough, generally people prefer not to have an enema as it feels like an invasion of privacy. Suppositories are torpedo-shaped pieces of glycerine placed in the rectum by using a finger and then retained while they melt and stimulate and lubricate the bowel. Overall, by far the best approach is to prevent constipation by having a good and varied diet and maintaining adequate fluid intake.

 Continence: key facts

- MND will not cause a person to become incontinent of urine or faeces

- People may encounter practical difficulties getting to and sitting on the toilet

- Many different aids are available to help people to remain clean and dry

- The community occupational therapist is the best person to advise on equipment

- Constipation is a common complaint for people living with MND and has many potential causes including change in activity, diet and ease of access to the lavatory

- A good diet and establishing a regular bowel routine are the key to preventing constipation and discomfort

- Various laxatives are available, and each works in a different way

- It is important to know the cause of the constipation in order to achieve relief

Should I give up work?

Being diagnosed with MND and the realization that it is a life-limiting disease can only be described as a totally devastating experience. An immediate tension is set up between a sense of loss for the future and a desire to maintain normality for the present. Each patient brings their own life goals and personality to bear on this situation, and the range of individual reactions is very varied. Some people are paralysed by a sense of hopelessness. Others wish to confront their situation head on. Our experience tells us that a period of adjustment to the new situation is required before most people are able to make major decisions. The journey ahead is not the one that was planned, but it need not be without rewards. By reflecting on what is important to us as individuals and what we wish to achieve, it is possible to give some structure to our life goals. One of the earliest thoughts that occurs to people is whether to stop working. For some people, work is simply defined as a means to an end, a way of providing life's necessities. For others, a job is an integral part of personal identity, in which case suddenly stopping work would be removing an important aspect of who we are. In addition, except for those with income protection policies or generous company sickness schemes allowing them to take early retirement, there may be a need to continue working for reasons of financial necessity. Our advice is that for most patients at the stage of initial diagnosis, there is no need to make decisions in a hurry. Take time to get advice from members of the care team and from the neurologist about the pace of change of the disease. While some people will want to redirect the emotional and physical energy involved in working towards time spent at home, travelling or pursuing hobbies, for others continuing to work is an important part of coping with MND.

When should I stop driving?

The Driver and Vehicle Licensing Authority (DVLA), and equivalent bodies in other countries, exists to regulate the right to hold a driving licence. There are a large body of rules surrounding the different types of driving licence in relation to various medical conditions. In some situations, such as loss of consciousness due to epilepsy, there is an automatic requirement to stop driving. With MND and other conditions in which disability accumulates rather slowly, there is no specific law that determines when people should stop driving. Neither is it the case that the decision is, strictly speaking, a medical one. Every driver who enters a motor vehicle bears an individual responsibility to be in full control of that vehicle. A failure to do so would be seen in law as a potentially serious offence. The problem arises that because disability develops in a piecemeal fashion in MND, and at the beginning of the illness function may be well maintained, the exact moment when a safe driver becomes a potentially unsafe one may be difficult to gauge. There is no simple answer to this conundrum, but there are a couple of elements of human behaviour related to driving which are worth bearing in mind.

We, especially men, generally overestimate our driving skills, and it is important to listen to those around us, family and friends, who will be sensitive to changes in our driving performance. Furthermore, because in the modern age, driving is intrinsically linked to our sense of personal freedom, many people suffer a loss of self-esteem when they realize they must stop driving. For those living in rural areas, who are dependent on motor transport for their social network, this is a particularly difficult issue. The wrong approach is to wait until an accident or near miss, however minor, occurs as a signal for change. Somehow one has to maintain a strong sense of personal insight and surveillance that enables a realistic assessment of one's own skills as a driver. As a minimum, at the time of diagnosis, patients with any significant neurological disease such as MND should inform their insurers and the DVLA of the diagnosis. This will not result in an instruction from these bodies that you should stop driving. The DVLA is likely to write to your neurologist for confirmation of your diagnosis and of the degree of physical disability. Generally, our advice is that if you begin to doubt your own ability to drive or if close family members are expressing concern, this is the time to stop. Occasionally, where there is doubt or dispute about fitness to drive, it is possible to arrange an appointment with a specialist driving assessor, who can also suggest adaptations to vehicles as appropriate. It is generally easier for them to provide useful advice for patients with stable conditions leading to disability, such as stroke, or very slowly progressive MND. In patients with typical forms of MND, if concerns about driving are being seriously raised, it is generally appropriate to stop driving altogether.

What is the best approach to planning changes to the environment?

The impact of MND changes with the different stages of the illness. Remaining in control imposes the need to make decisions and consider choices about changes to the home environment, often at a time when the natural impulse is to try and maintain a sense of normality. Should you move house or adapt the one you are currently living in? Is it a good idea to plan a stair lift, a 'through-floor' lift or move the bedroom downstairs? These decisions can be overwhelming, especially if many decision points occur simultaneously. The key to remaining in control is being able to make informed choices. When considering adaptations to the home, it is important to think carefully about the length of time the work will take. It is critical that the work occurs at a time when it will have the maximum impact on well-being. Employing builders, drawing up plans and obtaining planning permission potentially takes many months. Therefore, the best solution will depend on individual factors, including the type of disability and the pace of change of the disease. The community OT is trained to consider each person's individual circumstances and disability, assist them in navigating the process of home adaptation and advise on grants to help pay towards the work.

As the disease progresses, it may become more difficult to carry out certain tasks. However there are many different types of specialist equipment which are designed to enable people living with MND to remain as active and independent for as long as possible:

◆ Hand rails

◆ Aids to help get in and out of the bath

◆ Raised lavatory seats

◆ Perching stools

◆ Mobile arm supports

◆ Riser recliner chairs

◆ Bed elevators

◆ Pillow lifters

A team of health care professionals dedicated to supporting patients with motor weakness can do much which may improve quality of life and help people maximize their function in a difficult situation. However, interventions have to be rapid, and most health systems are simply not responsive enough to individual need at present. Mobile arm supports (MAS), also known as balanced forearm orthoses, balanced linkage feeders or ball-bearing arm supports, are a good example (Fig. 5.1). Originally developed in the USA in the 1930s to enable patients with polio to maximize upper limb strength, they can be used to aid eating, page turning, accessing the computer, painting, drawing and writing. Figure 5.1 demonstrates the use of the MAS to help in eating. The carefully engineered cantilevered system removes the mechanical disadvantage imposed by the weight of the arm to translate greatly reduced muscle power into large movements.

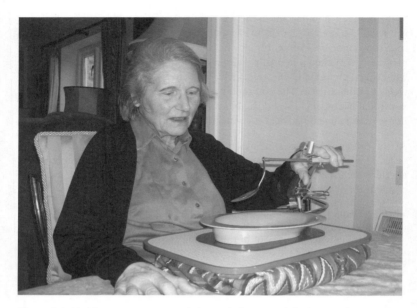

Figure 5.1 Mobile arm supports can help maximize strength in the arms by removing the force of gravity.

Timing is the key to successful use of MAS. Attempts to introduce them too early to people with good arm function result in failure because their relevance is not clear. Similarly, if there is too much delay in introduction so that there has been a long period of loss of use of the arms, people rarely manage to readapt. Early indications that MAS may be of benefit include resting the arm on the edge of the table and using it as a pivot to pick up food, stooping the head down low to meet the hand, as well as eating very slowly and tiring quickly. Our experience is that if a person with significant arm weakness has already accepted being fed by someone else, then they are unlikely to use a MAS to feed themselves.

Ankle supports can be useful if there is any weakness in the lower leg which results in not being able to raise the toe fully while walking ('foot drop'), which can lead to tripping. In MND these are often useful for a limited period and so 'off the shelf' supports which go down the back of the leg and under the feet are adequate. 'Made to measure' ankle supports can be provided by the local Orthotic Department, to which a GP, neurologist or physiotherapist can refer you.

Walking aids such as sticks and crutches can create psychological problems by confronting people with the reality that life is no longer normal, increasing the sense that one can no longer hide from others the fact that 'something is not right' and by representing a landmark in the progression of disability and a reminder that the disease is progressing. For these reasons, many people with MND are resistant to using walking aids. This is entirely understandable, but it is always better to avoid falls which, as well as risking serious injury, can lead to a loss of dignity and self-esteem. We often recommend that people initially try using a walker's stick, available from camping shops, which look less 'medical' and is therefore not noticed by others. It is important that advice is sought from an OT or physiotherapist to ensure that the correct aid is used and the risk of injury is minimized.

The idea of wheelchairs engenders mixed emotions in people living with MND. The acquisition of a wheelchair is sometimes regarded as an admission of failure or 'giving in' to disability and something that will hasten decline because the muscles are no longer being used. People fear the day that they use a wheelchair as a significant and ominous marker that MND is defeating them. In reality, use of a wheelchair is very often best considered at a time when walking function is still maintained. Initially a chair may be reserved just for outings that require longer distances as a way of conserving energy. It should be viewed positively as a way of 'getting from A to B' with ease and safety. It is critical to get specialist advice from an OT who will work closely with the local wheelchair service to advise, measure and supply the most appropriate chair. Depending on local funding arrangements, it may be possible to part-fund a more sophisticated chair according to individual needs and preferences. Wheelchairs must give adequate support to prevent complications such as pain in the neck, shoulders and arms, or a sore bottom.

Some people may develop weak neck muscles, making it difficult to hold the head up, or experience pain in the neck or shoulders. A neck support can offer some comfort. Like most pieces of equipment, there are many different types, and specialist advice is necessary. Collars and supports specially designed for neck weakness due to MND are available through physiotherapists and OTs.

How can I get a comfortable night's sleep?

Having a poor night's sleep can have a detrimental effect on well-being the following day. It can make carrying out the most minor of tasks tiring. Being awake through the night while others sleep can feel very lonely and demoralizing, and can be a time when our worst fears about living with MND come into people's consciousness. Therefore, it is essential that bed comfort is considered a high priority. The community OT and District Nurse will be able to give advice. They will consider the following:

◆ How will the person living with MND get up stairs to bed?

◆ Is it important for the person living with MND to remain in their double bed?

◆ A discussion may take part about an electronically operated 'hospital'-type bed called a 'profiling bed'. The head end is raised by the push of a button. Some beds also have an elevating knee section. This enables the person to move their position independently through the night. The switches can be adapted to increase sensitivity to touch or to be activated by the strongest part of the body if necessary.

◆ The height of the bed to enable easy access. If it is too low it can make getting to a standing position a strain.

◆ The position of the bed. Is it against a wall? Is there enough room to manoeuvre a wheelchair or commode?

The mattress is an important factor. People who have to lie in one position for any length of time may become prone to sore areas referred to as pressure sores. The areas of the body which are at most risk are at bony prominences such as the bottom of the spine, buttocks, hips, heels, elbows and shoulder blades. Pressure, usually from a bed or wheelchair, reduces circulation to the vulnerable parts of the body, depriving tissue of oxygen and other nutrients, and irreversible damage and tissue death can occur. Though the affected tissue may die in as little as 12 hours, the injury may not be apparent for days or even weeks. Pressure sores can develop quickly, progress rapidly and are often difficult to heal. In some cases, the pressure that cuts off the circulation comes from unlikely sources: the rivets and thick seams in jeans, crumbs in bed, wrinkled clothing or sheets, even perspiration, which can soften skin, making it more vulnerable to injury. An early warning sign of pressure damage is a red patch on the skin, which may feel slightly sore or itchy. Do not ignore this, if left it will develop in into a sore. Pressure sores are preventable by a regular change of position, ideally at least every 30 minutes when sitting and every 2 hours while in bed. The use of pressure-relieving cushions and mattresses will contribute towards the reduction of pressure sores and enhance comfort.

There are many different types of mattress. 'Memory foam' mattresses mould to your shape and give support and aid in pressure relieving by distributing body weight evenly. People report that they are very comfortable and reduce the number of times they need to turn at night. However, once on the mattress, the body sinks into it slightly which does make turning more difficult. An 'alternating air mattress' is made up of separate cells through which air circulates at varying intervals. Thus the cells of the mattress inflate and deflate at different times, relieving the pressure on the body every few minutes. Air mattresses make a slight noise due to the air pump, but this does not interfere with sleep and can even be quite soothing. Water beds work by relieving pressure that is exerted directly on the bony prominences. In addition to feeling a little unusual compared with a conventional bed, it is not possible to raise the head end with water mattresses to enable a person living with MND to sit up. Getting on and off them can also be tricky. The OT and District Nurse are the best professionals to advise which mattress is the most appropriate, and will have a supply of mattresses for trial.

Summary

In this chapter, we have tried to emphasize that, although MND is a progressive condition, there is much that can be done by the care team to help people who are living with MND. Interventions have the most value if they are tailored to individual needs and life goals, and if they are available in a timely fashion.

6

Special situations in motor neuron disease

Inherited motor neuron disease

Genetic disease is a very complex area of medicine, and the information contained in this chapter, while it is intended to be a helpful guide, should not replace the need to get specialist advice. We strongly advise anyone who thinks that they may be at risk of inherited MND to seek specialist counselling through the normal medical services.

What are the differences between inherited and non-inherited forms of MND?

As discussed in earlier chapters, a small proportion (between 5 and 10 per cent) of patients with MND have a family history of the disease. In this situation, the MND is said to be **familial.** In one-fifth of these familial cases, scientists have identified genetic errors (mutations) in a gene called superoxide dismutase 1 (SOD1). This is currently the only genetic test available for familial MND and in the 80 per cent of people with inherited MND who do not have confirmed SOD1 mutations we are unable to test other family members. Apart from a family history, individual patients with familial MND are otherwise indistinguishable from patients with non-inherited or so-called **sporadic** MND. In fact, when large numbers of familial MND patients have been studied, it is clear that on average the disease comes on about 10 years earlier, though there is still a wide range of ages at which people can be affected. The same variation in disease seen in sporadic MND, with different degrees of involvement of upper and lower motor neurons, is also seen in familial MND. It is also possible to have quite different patterns within the same family, suggesting that a single type of genetic mutation can lead to different forms of MND. These facts provide some support for the idea that inherited MND, caused by mutations in a single gene, and sporadic MND, where the cause is unknown, are still related in terms of the way that the disease develops in the nervous system. This is important for MND research, since a very high proportion of scientific effort is currently devoted to understanding the cause of motor neuron death in cases of familial MND caused by mutations in the SOD1 gene, and in testing potential drugs in the mouse model of SOD1-related MND. Much hope is invested in drugs which appear to show an effect in the SOD1 mouse. On the other hand, neuropathologists recognize subtle differences in the brain and spinal cord of people with familial MND which may suggest that there are differences in the basic mechanisms of these diseases. Furthermore, so far, the SOD1 animal model has not proved to be a good screening tool for new drugs. A number of substances which have slowed progression in this animal model have failed to show the same effect in clinical trials in patients with sporadic MND. At present the relationship between familial and sporadic MND at the pathological level remains uncertain. In terms of symptom management for practical purposes, the diseases are managed in the same way.

What are the implications of having an inherited form of MND?

One thing that is profoundly different for people with familial MND is the experience of coping with the information that other members of the family are at risk of the same disease. This can sometimes be a very difficult experience and almost always requires counselling from a specialist team composed of a clinical geneticist, who is a doctor specializing in genetically inherited disease, and a neurologist who is an expert in MND. Although genetic errors leading to human diseases are due to random biological events which are beyond our control, it is common for a patient with familial MND to feel a sense of guilt and responsibility for potentially passing on the risk of MND.

As with many aspects of MND, the first stage in conquering the psychological impact of the disease is to have a good knowledge of what inheritance means. At the time of the initial consultation with a neurologist specializing in MND, it is usual for a detailed family history to be taken. To help explain the issues, we have made up the Jones family. Sarah Jones has presented to the neurology clinic, where a diagnosis of MND has been made. A full family history was taken and is represented in the diagram below.

◆ Is this a family with familial MND? As well as Sarah, there are others who appear to have had a neurological problem. Not uncommonly, it is difficult to be certain of the exact cause of death of people in generations past such as Sarah's grandfather John Smith. This is partly because access to specialists was less good in the past and people with MND did not always have a firm diagnosis, but also because medical matters were not discussed so openly, either between doctor and patient or within families. The Jones family are unsure if John Smith had MND but they strongly suspect that he did.

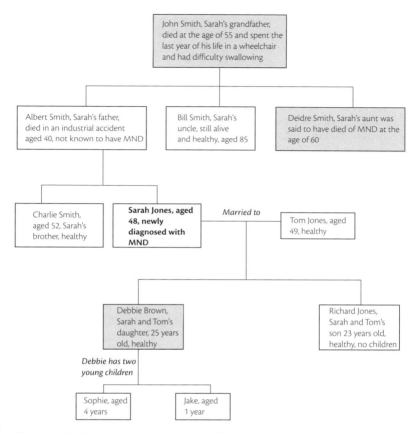

Figure 6.1 Is this a family with inherited MND?

To a neurologist, the history of someone with mobility problems, swallowing difficulties and an illness that resulted in death within a few years is strongly suggestive of MND. Sarah's aunt Deidre's death certificate clearly states that she died from MND. Therefore, it looks very much like three people in three separate generations have developed MND. This is a clear indication that an abnormal or mutant form of a gene is being passed through the family and causing MND.

◆ Why has Sarah's uncle, Bill Smith, not developed MND by now? The complete number of genes that we possess, approximately 25 000, is collectively referred to as our genome, and each gene is represented twice. We inherit one copy from each parent. Therefore, in inherited forms of MND such as in the Jones family, the 'MND-causing gene' exists in a normal copy and an abnormal or mutant copy. An affected individual such as John Smith can pass on either the abnormal copy or the normal copy. John Smith's wife will possess two normal copies and will therefore always pass on a normal gene to her children. So, it should follow that each of John Smith's children would have a 50 per cent risk of inheriting the abnormal gene from him. The most likely reason that Bill has not developed MND is simply that he has inherited the normal copy of the gene from his father rather than the abnormal one. Another less likely possibility is that Bill does indeed possess the abnormal copy of the gene but for some reason the disease has not developed. Perhaps other genetic and non-genetic factors have in some way protected Bill. This occasionally happens in MND.

◆ Why did Sarah's father not develop MND? Sarah's father died at a relatively young age from an accident. Given that in this family the typical age at which MND develops is after the late 40s, then Albert Smith is most likely to have died from another cause before the age at which he would have suffered from MND. In order for Sarah to have MND, she must have inherited the faulty gene from her father.

◆ What is the risk to Sarah's brother, Charlie Smith? Some people make the mistake of thinking that because one person in a generation inherited an abnormal gene that the next person will naturally inherit the normal copy. In fact, each time a person passes on their genetic material the probability that either of the two copies will be passed on is exactly 50 per cent. It is just like tossing a coin. Another common misconception is that people in a family who are superficially alike ('she takes after her father rather than her mother') share all of the same characteristics. Just because Charlie Smith is just like his father in appearance and personality, his risk of inheriting the faulty MND gene is 50 per cent, no more, no less. The fact that he is 52, and Sarah has developed the disease at 48, does not mean that he has passed the age where MND may occur. Even within the same family the age at which genetic disease can develop can vary considerably. Aunt Deidre, for example, died from MND when she was 60.

◆ What is the risk to Sarah's children? Because Sarah has MND, she must carry one abnormal gene copy and one normal gene copy. Therefore, each of her children is at 50 per cent risk of carrying the disease gene variant. The actual risk of getting MND in this situation is usually quoted as being slightly less than 50 per cent because of the occasional cases, mentioned above, of gene carriers who do not manifest the disease.

◆ What is the risk to Sarah's grandchildren? This is a little more complex. If each of Sarah's children has a 50 per cent chance of carrying the disease gene, then each of her grandchildren has half that chance, 25 per cent, of also being a carrier.

What should I tell my children?

The emergence of a genetic disease within families can be a source of great anxiety, especially when young members of the family may not be fully able to absorb the implications. Given that this information may also become apparent at the very time when the family is coming to terms with the news that someone is suffering from MND, it can sometimes provoke a crisis. People naturally respond to this in a variety of different ways, ranging from complete openness to a wish to conceal difficult news in order to protect loved ones. These are difficult decisions, and it is not the job of doctors to confront people with information which they are not ready to cope with or dictate to patients and their families how to behave. However, experience generally tells us that when these issues are not openly discussed, resentment may build up and this may create a barrier preventing the mutual support that is so necessary if family members are to help each other cope with a difficult disease like MND.

As adults, we frequently underestimate the level to which children understand the impact of illness and even the nature of inheritance. Genetics and other biological topics are much more the currency of education and everyday life than in the past. We generally recommend that the most healthy approach to talking to children about both MND in general and inherited MND in particular is to respond to their questions with openness and honesty. However, the child should in some respects dictate the pace at which this information is offered, and confronting children with too much information too soon may generate undue anxiety and confusion.

Should other family members be tested?

At the present time, MND is not a curable disease. If there were treatments which significantly modify the disease process, it would follow that intervening at the earliest possible time would give people the most benefit. In this situation, it would be in the interests of those at risk to know their genetic status once they become adults and to be followed up in a specialist clinic so that drugs could be given at the early stage of disease or, ideally, even before the disease begins. Therefore, at the current time, someone who is the first-degree relative (parent, sibling or child) of a patient with inherited MND, and has a 50 per cent risk of inheriting the abnormal gene, is unlikely to gain very much from knowing their own status. Remember, that in any case this is only possible in the 20 per cent of families who have SOD1 mutations. Some people who are at 50 per cent risk of MND feel that they wish to know their own status as it would affect their own choice whether to have children. While this seems on the face of it to be a reasonable view, the decision whether or not to test people must be based on the implications for the individual currently at risk, not on future generations. Although ideas about preventing the birth of those carrying genetic disease may vary from one culture to another and also throughout different periods of human history, it is currently the case that most people would not want to avoid the birth of children at risk of developing genetic disease 40–50 years into the future, a time when there will certainly be a much greater prospect of curative treatments than at present.

 Patient's perspective

Barry is 45 years old and comes to the MND clinic for advice. Barry's mother Joan, his aunt Catherine and his sister Amanda have all died of MND, which in each case came on in their mid-40s and led to their death within 3 years. Barry has been told that a laboratory in the North-West of England identified mutations in his family and he is very keen to be tested. We contacted the laboratory and were able to confirm that Barry's relatives with MND carried a mutation in the SOD1 gene. Should Barry be offered testing?

A joint consultation with a clinical geneticist and a neurologist specializing in MND was organized for Barry. Given that he had lived with the knowledge that he was at risk of MND for more than 20 years, we wanted to explore his motivation for being tested at this time. It emerged that he was engaged to be married and his fiancée had insisted that he undergo testing before the wedding. Barry appeared to be relaxed about the consequences of finding out that he might be carrying the gene mutation, and said that he would 'take the news whether it was good or bad'. However, we were concerned that Barry's wish to be tested was being driven by the wishes of others and asked him to spend a month reconsidering his decision to be tested.

He returned to clinic and, despite further counselling, was firm in his decision to have the genetic test.

He tested positive for the mutation. Soon afterwards his fiancée called off the engagement.

Lessons:

❖ Patients at risk of genetic diseases such as familial MND have the right to be tested, but health care professionals must help the patient consider the full implications of both a positive and a negative test.

❖ People with a family history of MND in first-degree relatives live with the knowledge that they have a 50 per cent risk of developing the disease. If they are still healthy but test positive for a mutation, they have moved from a 50 per cent risk to one that is close to 100 per cent. They should consider very carefully, before agreeing to testing, that they are prepared for this possibility.

MND in young people

Approximately 10 per cent of people with MND develop the disease below the age of 40 years. Fewer than 1 per cent of patients are below the age of 25, and MND, as we would normally recognize it, is almost unheard of before the age of 20. This is part of the biological variation in the way that MND behaves, but there are some particular issues that arise when young people are affected.

Is MND affecting young people a different disease?

In most respects, the pattern of disease in young people is not significantly different and all of the different clinical variants have been described in younger people. Taken overall, younger people are more likely to have a slower disease progression and to have lower motor neuron predominant disease. However, as with MND in general, it is difficult to apply these generalizations to individuals, and there is great variation. There is nothing to suggest that MND is fundamentally a different disease in young people, but the trends in disease pattern might suggest that some of the complex factors thought to be involved in MND susceptibility are acting in a stronger way than others. For example, if in general MND is an age-dependent process, the reason that it comes on early in some individuals might relate to the operation of a few strong genetic factors. There is absolutely no reason to believe that sporadic MND (i.e. where there is no family history of a similar condition) coming on at an unusually young age will be passed on, however. In the absence of a family history, the risk to first-degree relatives is still very small.

There are a number of other diseases of the motor neuron which can present in younger people and, given the rarity of MND in the under-40 age group, neurologists must think carefully and will probably perform a greater number of diagnostic tests in order to exclude these. Certain genetic disorders which in the early stages may mimic MND present in this age group. Overall, people with younger onset MND are more likely to have investigations such as lumbar puncture and even to have a trial of therapies such as IVIG (intravenous immunoglobulin) in order to make sure that a treatable disorder is not being missed.

What are the effects on young children of having a parent with MND?

The response to receiving a diagnosis of MND is a very individual one, whatever the age of the patient. However, it is generally true that people in their 80s may have come to terms with the fact that their lifespan is limited. In contrast, the development of a terminal illness in the 30s or 40s will inevitably seem like a 'bolt from the blue' and there will be a sense of shock which is transmitted to every aspect of the person's life. On an individual level, the person with MND undergoes a very real bereavement process with a strong sense of loss for an anticipated future (see Chapter 3). In young onset MND, there may be very strong feelings of guilt about the effect of the disease on partners (who may have to work, look after children and care for a sick person).

One of the greatest challenges for young parents coping with a new diagnosis of MND is what to tell the children. Generally speaking, children are very sensitive to a change in the atmosphere at home. Attempting to maintain a sense of normality by denying that there is a problem usually leads to a disturbance to children's equilibrium. Children are both very sensitive to change and, compared with adults, better able to absorb it. We generally recommend an open attitude where children's questions are answered in a straightforward and honest way. Information is best delivered in a graded way without necessarily confronting children with the long-term consequences of what is happening, until they are ready to ask those questions. Otherwise one can create a sense of great foreboding without the child having the necessary knowledge to come to some resolution.

The painful issue of very young children growing up perhaps never knowing one of their parents is a difficult one. We sometimes help and encourage people to make a video legacy for their children.

Cognitive impairment

Is it ever a feature of MND?

It has always been known that very rarely, perhaps in 2–3 per cent of patients, MND is associated with a form of dementia in which language and behaviour are affected. This may begin either before the usual features of MND develop or at the same time, and is frequently a severe problem, sometimes more disabling than the weakness. It was otherwise believed that the other 98 per cent of patients have completely normal mental (or what neurologists call 'cognitive') function. However, in recent years our thinking has evolved. It has become clear that a significant proportion (30–40 per cent) of patients with MND have some difficulties in cognitive tasks such as planning and decision making, emotional control and some aspects of language. In many cases, this is mild and not a significant issue for the person with MND. However, occasionally it is a prominent part of the clinical picture and requires some management in its own right. Even when cognitive changes are mild, it is usually helpful for the family and carers of the person with MND to be fully informed about this to avoid misunderstanding the individual's change in behaviour and the resulting frustration and upset which can arise in everyday life. The person with MND may be completely unaware of the problem and, when it is explained, may simply respond with indifference. Although it is difficult to generalize completely, and more work needs to be done to study the problem, our experience is that mild cognitive impairment is usually detectable early in the disease course and tends not to develop as a late feature. Therefore, the majority of patients with MND should not fear that important mental faculties such as judgement and the ability to make independent decisions will be impaired. However, this relatively recent realization that some patients have mild to moderate impairments can have important implications in decision planning and in drawing up advance directives.

 Patient's perspective

Brian is 64 years old and has had a diagnosis of MND for about a year. His wife Sheila is becoming progressively frustrated. If she pops out to the shops and leaves Brian alone, he just sits in a chair watching TV, even though he is still capable of tending to his garden and doing simple household chores. On several occasions he has failed to pass on important telephone messages. Brian does not seem aware that this is a change in behaviour, which would be unusual for someone who used to be an accountant and for whom making decisions was an everyday part of life. In many ways, Brian is the same affable person he always was. Friends and relatives have commented that he is being very brave about having MND and seems to be coping well, but Sheila is worried that he is in denial or even severely depressed. Things come to a head when her frustration leads to a row and, for the first time in their 28 years of married life, Brian lashes out and tries to hit her.

Assessment in the MND clinic by a psychologist reveals that Brian is not depressed but is showing some impairments on psychological tests in what is called 'executive' function; that part of our mental faculties to do with complex thinking such as judgement, motivation, etc. Once the problem has been explained to Sheila and she realizes that this is part of Brian's MND, they are able to continue, with Sheila making some allowances. The psychological aspects of Brian's disease never really got worse with time and was never the dominating feature for him or Sheila.

There are many reasons why someone with MND may show signs of withdrawal and disengagement from their situation. While mild cognitive impairment can be the explanation, it is important to rule out other possibilities. Depression (discussed in a previous chapter) can occur in people with MND and, in addition to low mood, can manifest as apathy, lack of motivation and difficulty in making decisions. Weak breathing muscles leading to disturbed oxygen exchange during sleep can cause mental clouding and sleepiness during the day. Sometimes it is simply that the person with MND is responding to the difficulties of the disease by 'switching off' and withdrawing into a kind of inner world. Psychologists sometimes call this an 'adjustment reaction'. A full psychological assessment may help in differentiating between these different causes, but occasionally a trial of an antidepressant is justified in an effort to see if treating low mood can improve well-being.

Living with very slowly progressive disease

Throughout this book we have placed great emphasis on the variability in disease progression that is seen with MND. Approximately 10 per cent of patients live with MND for more than 10 years. At the beginning of the illness it may be very difficult for doctors to predict a slowly progressive course, and many patients who live for a longer than the expected time have gone through a period of adjusting to a shortened lifespan before if it becomes apparent that they will live for decades.

 Patient's perspective

Mary is now in her late 50s and has had MND for 25 years. When she first developed symptoms and signs of the disease it seemed to be progressing in a fairly typical way and she was told to prepare for the likelihood that she would live for 2–3 years. While this was a devastating blow for someone in their 30s, with time she adjusted to the situation. She was discharged from neurological care, and rehabilitation specialists arranged for various support measures at home. After 2–3 years it became clear that, while Mary was unable to care for herself independently, her disease was progressing very slowly. After 5 years she had lost the ability to speak, was confined to a wheelchair and needed full-time care as she lived alone. After a few years more, she developed a relationship with a man who had been involved in engineering some aids in her home. After 8 years of marriage they divorced and Mary resumed her life alone with full-time carers. She developed breast cancer 6 years ago which was successfully treated. When Mary reflects on her life, she has a mixture of emotions. On the one hand, she continues to lead a busy life with lots of social interaction. On the other hand, she has periods of gloom, anger and even despair at her situation. She has expressed anger directed at the doctors who told her she would only live for a couple of years.

Is very slowly progressive MND a different disease?

Why do some people with MND, such as the famous example of Professor Stephen Hawking, have a very extended lifespan? As with most other aspects of the disease, the simple answer is that we do not yet understand the biological basis of this variability. When pathologists have studied the spinal cord and brain of people with MND that has gone on for many years, there are few clues. In many respects, the disease looks the same under the microscope. Most MND specialists tend to agree that the great variability in the course of MND reflects some intrinsic biological differences between individuals which quite possibly has a genetic basis. According to this model, some people carry genetic variants which act to slow down the disease process. An alternative explanation is that slowly progressive MND is a different disease with different causes. Because, in the context of MND overall, these patients are relatively rare, it is not an easy problem to study and will require cooperation between large groups of clinics who can collect data and DNA from many patients. If we could understand why some people have a slowly progressive course, this might well allow us to design or choose therapies which will slow the disease in people with more typical forms of MND.

Can the mental attitude of patients have an effect on the disease course?

Many people with MND have said to us that they intend to beat the disease by using the power of their own personality and will to 'think positively'. We have learned to appreciate that some people are endowed with an extraordinary strength of will and that this can certainly make a difference. There is also some limited evidence that people who are highly motivated to continue living with MND will actively seek out specialist centres and make use of every possible management option such as PEG and NIV. However, taken overall, there is nothing to suggest that the reason that some people live for decades is due to mental attitude. It is particularly important that people with typical MND are not left feeling that they are contributing to their own decline because they are unable to be more positive. MND is a potentially demoralizing disease, and it is perfectly normal to feel a sense of powerlessness from time to time.

How do people with slowly progressive MND cope?

For people without neurological disability, the idea that one might find oneself in a state of immobility, where all daily needs require the help of others and where communication is very limited, is unthinkable and perhaps the stuff of nightmares. This view arises largely from a process of catastrophic thinking where we can only imagine an immediate transition from complete health to total disability. While this is what happens to people who have suffered major trauma from a car crash, the process of adapting to disability in slowly progressive MND is quite a different journey. MND, whichever form if takes, is a disease which will be 'mapped' on to the pre-existing personality of the sufferer. This means that we have witnessed an extraordinary range of individual responses to increasing disability. In fact, most people with slowly progressive MND develop coping mechanisms which allow them to adapt to each stage of the disease. Generally, the most difficult psychological disturbance arises when people are unable to stop themselves from projecting into the future to a time when they have a different set of problems from the current ones.

7

Participating in research

Introduction

Because MND is a relatively rare disease compared with many others seen in a neurological clinic, most patients will be referred to specialist MND centres (such as those supported by the MNDA in the UK). Neurologists specializing in MND frequently lead or participate in research into the causes of the disease. Many patients with MND are highly motivated to contribute to the research effort and will often travel great distances to participate in clinical trials. This is naturally in the hope of getting some benefit, but also an expression of willingness to help future sufferers with MND. The purpose of this chapter is to provide some background information about what is involved in research participation and some of the pros and cons of being a research subject.

How are research projects organized?

It is recognized that people participating in research projects are potentially vulnerable. Experience from crimes against humanity committed during the Second World War led to the Declaration of Helsinki, which enshrines the principle that research can only proceed in a morally acceptable way with the informed consent of research subjects. Untoward events such as side effects from drugs can occur, or research may simply be physically or psychologically stressful. For this reason, before a research project can get underway, it has to be passed by a **Research Ethics Committee**, a group of doctors, other health care professionals and lay representatives appointed by a hospital to scrutinize research. This process involves a written application from the researchers in which the research is described in detail. Among the questions that have to be addressed by the Ethics Committee are:

* Why the research needs to be done. Is the question being asked by the researchers an important one? Will an answer lead to potential benefit for patients? Curiosity on the part of the researchers is not sufficient justification.

* Does the proposed project have the power to answer the question being asked? Unfortunately many trials of new treatments use insufficient numbers of patients to detect a statistically significant effect. These trials are sometimes justified on the grounds of testing tolerability or safety, but all too often it simply reflects poor design and does not move our knowledge forward at all.

* What will happen to participants? The Ethics Committee has to be reassured that the research subjects will not undergo unjustified discomfort or potential harm, and that the subjects are correctly informed about what will happen.

* What risks are associated with the project? Given that the side effects of drugs or other interventions are not completely understood until there is considerable clinical experience and many patients have been treated, the Ethics Committee can only ensure that these risks are minimized. There can never be a guarantee that the research will be entirely risk free.

* Who are the people doing the research? The Committee concerns itself with ascertaining that the researchers are legitimate: that they are *bone fide* medical experts who have the knowhow and facilities to conduct the research properly.

* Will the researchers or research participants get any material benefit (financial or otherwise) from conducting the research? Drug trials are often carried out in hospitals under a contract from a commercial sponsor such as a pharmaceutical company. In this situation, the salaries of members of the research team may be supported by money from commercial sources. It is important to ensure that the income from such sources is reasonable and fully accounted for, and that patients are not being exploited for the profit of individuals or organizations. In other situations, the researchers lead the trial but funding is obtained by applying for grants from charities or bodies such as the UK Medical Research Council. In this case, the application will be carefully reviewed by fellow scientists (so-called 'peer review') and there is less chance of research funds being used inappropriately.

A full application to a Research Ethics Committee is very time consuming. While some researchers feel that the very high level of scrutiny and the considerable amount of paperwork required by the Ethics Committee can create barriers to research, there is general consensus that it is important to protect patients and to prevent the kind of human rights abuses that have occurred in less liberal times in human history.

In addition to seeking ethical approval, researchers must obtain funding to support the costs of research. It will not be a surprise to learn that conducting research is an expensive activity, but most people do not realize just how expensive it is. To run a single project studying the progress of MND using sophisticated MRI scanning, for example, will cost in the region of £100 000 per year. A typical trial of a new drug in a disease such as MND will cost millions of pounds. The annual budget of the Medical Research Council, the main government source of medical research funding, was approximately £450 million in 2004. This falls very far short of what is required to support modern medical research in the UK and is a fraction (about 0.5 per cent) of the total annual NHS budget for delivering medical care. There are other sources of funding such as the MNDA and other charities, but overall there is a feeling among scientists that progress in medical research would be helped by an increase in funding. It does not necessarily follow, however, that throwing large sums of money at a difficult problem like MND will lead to a solution overnight.

How are drug trials designed?

Drug trials in a disease such as MND are a major undertaking for both the subjects and the investigators. In order to decide if a drug has a useful clinical effect, it is necessary to conduct the trial according to very specific design principles with a method called a **randomized controlled trial**.

1. One group of patients takes the active drug under investigation. A **control** group, identical in every way to the subjects taking the active drug, are given a **placebo**, an inactive substance which looks and tastes identical to the drug. It is critical that both groups are matched with respect to age, sex and severity of disease. For example, it is generally true that older patients with MND survive for a shorter time than younger patients. A trial in which the group taking active drug were on average younger than the group taking placebo could therefore lead to the false conclusion that the drug improved survival. In reality, this group would have survived overall for longer anyway because they were younger.

2. Subjects are **randomized** to receive either active drug or a placebo. Randomization is important because if researchers were allowed to choose who received drug and who received placebo, it is possible that this would bias the outcome of the trial by the investigators unconsciously allocating less severely affected patients to the treatment group. True randomization means that the chance of each patient receiving active drug is exactly 50 per cent.

3. Neither subject nor investigator must know whether an individual is on active drug or placebo. This is known as **blinding**. Patients who suspect they are taking active drugs tend to report improvements in symptoms. It becomes impossible to know if this is just a reflection of their natural desire to see an improvement or a real effect of the drug. Similarly, investigators may be biased in their assessment of improvement if they know if a patient is on active drug or placebo. Blinding sometimes breaks down if the active drug has clear side effects (e.g. raising body temperature).

Another critical aspect of trial design relates to the number of patients involved. If the effect of a drug was so dramatic that it led to a complete cure of a disease and caused no ill effects, then once a small number of patients had been successfully treated it would be easy to argue that the drug should be immediately available to all patients with the disease. However, the effects we might anticpate with potential therapies for MND at present are likely to be more modest. Almost all biological processes, and therefore all diseases, are subject to random fluctuations. No two patients will have exactly the same disease course. With small numbers of subjects, these fluctuations in the natural history of a disease can lead to chance differences between groups. Such chance effects are much less likely to occur if large numbers of patients are used. Before starting a trial, researchers model the possible effects they are expecting and calculate the number of patients they should include in each treatment group to avoid biases due to chance and to detect a real effect. This is known as a 'power calculation'. Only trials which are designed in this way are likely to produce a clear and reliable result. Unfortunately, many trials are underpowered and therefore do not produce a clear result.

What is it like to be a subject in a drug trial?

Most patients who volunteer for clinical trials research do so with a strong sense of hope and optimism that some good will come of their efforts. The history of MND drug trial research over the last 20 years, however, is a story of many false dawns and few positive results. It is therefore inevitable that many patients will have become disillusioned along the way. On the other hand, there is no doubt that participating in trials for a disease in which treatment options are currently limited offers an opportunity to be proactive and to feel that one is 'doing something'.

Clinical trials in MND start with a screening examination. The purpose of this is to establish that the potential participant fits agreed criteria, with the aim of including patients with the typical ALS form of MND and excluding patients in whom the diagnosis of MND is in doubt and who may turn out to have other conditions. Including patients with other diagnoses would reduce the power of the study and potentially produce misleading results. While this seems justified, it does have the unfortunate effect of allowing regulatory authorities to claim that evidence from trials can only be applied to patients with 'typical ALS', potentially excluding use of drugs in people with more slowly progressive or atypical forms of MND such as PLS. Similarly, and probably less justified, is that most clinical trials to date have used an age limit of 70 or 75. In an age-dependent condition such as MND, this will exclude many potential participants and also lead to uncertainty about whether the drug is safe in the elderly population. Women of childbearing age are either excluded completely or must be using adequate methods of contraception as a condition of entry to the trial. This is because at the early stage of drug development it will be unclear whether the experimental drug could affect the developing embryo. Even if it is unlikely that women with MND would become pregnant, trial investigators have a serious responsibility to prevent the kind of medical tragedy that happened with the drug thalidomide in the 1960s, where many children were born with limb deformities due to exposure to the drug in the womb. In summary, screening will therefore exclude people who (1) have atypical forms of MND or might not have MND at all; (2) have taken drugs which could confound the effect of the trial drug (e.g. drugs with potential but unproven neuroprotective effects); (3) the elderly and women of childbearing age who might become pregnant; and (4) people with other illnesses affecting mobility and breathing which would interfere with the evaluation of the drug.

Once patients have been screened and found to fit the entry criteria, the next stage is **randomization**. This is the method whereby people are allocated to having either active drug or placebo. This is one of the most difficult aspects of clinical trial methodology for people to understand and accept. No one puts themselves forward for a clinical trial hoping to get allocated the placebo! Yet it is fundamental to understanding if a drug works to know that apparent benefit is not caused simply by participating in the trial. Similarly, we must be absolutely sure that we have a clear understanding of the potential harm that drugs can cause. Figure 7.1 is taken from a publication describing a clinical trial of a drug called topiramate in patients with MND. The trial showed no benefit from this drug, but it is interesting to note that both patients taking topiramate and patients taking placebo also complained of side effects. How can a placebo, which is by definition an inactive tablet, cause 13.4 per cent of people who took it to become nauseated? This is a powerful demonstration that, if directly questioned about non-specific symptoms such as tiredness, headache, nausea and mood disturbance, what emerges is a natural day-to-day variation in how we experience our body that could easily be misinterpreted as due to disease or a drug treatment. It is therefore critical that both the potential harm caused by drugs and also any treatment effects are compared with a placebo. Muscle strength and general well-being can both vary from day to day depending on our mood, how well we have slept, what we have eaten and even the weather. Both the treating doctor and the trial participant are naturally hoping that the trial drug will work. Patients in clinical trials are self-selected as highly motivated to get better. This alone can produce apparent improvements in function. Only when it is compared with placebo can we really be sure that a drug is both efficacious and safe.

When dealing with the assessment of drugs in which the anticipated treatment effect is relatively modest, such as extension of lifespan by months or a slowing

Table 2 Adverse events

	Total Occurrence N (%)	Topiramate n = 197	Placebo n = 97	*p* = Values
Anorexia	76 (25.9)	65 (33.0)	11 (11.3)	0.0001
Depression	67 (22.8)	55 (27.9)	12 (12.4)	0.003
Diarrhoea	42 (14.3)	34 (17.3)	8 (8.2)	0.05
Echymosis (bruising)	9 (3.1)	9 (4.7)	0 (0)	0.03
Kidney stones	18 (6.1)	18 (9.1)	0 (0)	0.001
Nausea	66 (22.2)	53 (26.9)	**13 (13.4)**	0.01
Paresthesia	32 (10.9)	27 (13.7)	5 (5.2)	0.03
Pulmonary embolism or Deep venous thrombosis	13 (4.4)	12 (6.1)	1 (1.0)	0.07
Thinking abnormalities	39 (13.2)	36 (18.3)	3 (3.1)	0.0002
Weight decrease	31 (10.5)	27 (13.7)	4 (4.1)	0.01

Values are number (%).
460 NEUROLOGY 61 August (2 of 2) 2003

Table 7.1 The placebo effect. In clinical trials, positive and negative symptoms are usually reported both by patients taking active drug and by those taking placebo.

of progress of the disease, large numbers of participants are required in order to provide enough statistical power. Therefore, each MND centre will be part of a large network involved in the trial which is likely to span several European countries or, in the USA, many clinics spread across the country. Currently, clinical trials tend to have in excess of 400 patients in each 'arm' (active drug or placebo) of the trial. If a drug had a dramatic effect, clearly fewer participants would be required. The large number of patients required also reflects the fact that we still do not have good measures of disease progression for MND. Measuring change, when the pattern and rate of progression are so variable, is not easy. Each measurement in use has its own problems. A popular approach is to use the ALS Functional Rating Scale (ALSFRS) which has been devised to take account of a range of measures of motor function (mobility, speech and swallowing, simple activities of daily living) and provides a reasonable correlation with overall disease progression. The ALSFRS has a maximum score of 40 points. However, it is not a linear scale, which means that the difference between 25 and 30, and 20 and 25 points is not necessarily the same. Therefore, if ALSFRS is the main outcome measure of the effect of a drug, complex statistics may be required to analyse the data. Another commonly used measure of disease progression is the rate of change of respiratory muscle function using vital capacity (VC, see Chapter 4, page 64). Although this also shows a reasonable correlation with disease progression, there are a significant number of patients in whom FVC is technically difficult to measure, and it is also subject to variation depending on who is performing the test. Some trials have used measurement of muscle strength combined across a range of muscle groups and then added together to make a combined muscle score. This is an attractive approach, but is even more open to variability between examiners.

Generally, trial participants are assessed at regular intervals with a repeat examination and an enquiry about symptoms and side effects. This may occur every 2–3 months and necessarily has to be a 'business-like' exercise in recording information, both about disease progression and about side effects, to produce a complete picture of drug safety. Therefore, it is in no way a replacement for the normal clinical care that people with MND should receive. Furthermore, at each trial visit, a blood sample will be taken to look for any evidence that the trial drug is causing harm, something that would not occur during routine MND outpatient visits.

What are the risks of taking part in drug trials?

Drugs that have a potentially beneficial biological effect can also do harm. It can never be assumed that a drug is safe until many thousands of patients have taken it. By definition, clinical trials are conducted at a time when only a small number of human subjects will have taken the drug, and so there is always an element of uncertainty regarding safety. Taking a drug in the context of a trial must therefore be assumed to carry more risk than taking a drug prescribed under normal circumstances. Despite this, clinical trials of new drugs have an excellent safety record. This is because any new compound produced by a pharmaceutical laboratory is first tested on animals to assess toxicity. Then, in so-called **Phase I** studies, healthy human volunteers are given the drug and assessed for signs of organ dysfunction and for how the body handles and eliminates the drug. **Phase II** studies are performed in larger groups, this time patients with the target disease, both to assess toxicity further and to look for evidence of efficacy. If the drug does not cause harm, it is usually necessary to perform larger **Phase III** studies to provide definitive evidence in favour or against benefit and to compare the drug with standard treatment. For example, it is all very well if a new drug is a good treatment for headache but we also need to know if it is any better than the treatments which are already available. This process of trying a drug in animals first, then healthy volunteers and finally in patients has proved to be a safe way to proceed. However, there are examples of drugs which seems safe for the majority of people, but which in certain individuals can cause serious or even fatal side effects. Most patients who enter clinical trials of new therapies for MND are willing to accept this small risk, knowing that they have a disease which is currently incurable and will ultimately shorten their life. However, as with every other aspect of clinical trials, it is critical that informed consent is freely given.

In summary, participating in a clinical trial involves extra visits to the hospital, extra blood samples and other tests which may be uncomfortable, the risk of unwanted side effects and a potential for loss of morale if it becomes clear that the drug does not work. On the other hand, there is little doubt that the extra scrutiny accorded to patients in clinical trials in MND has led to a general improvement in care and in how we measure changes in function as the disease progresses. Many patients have gained something from their participation and derive a positive feeling that they are contributing to the battle to find treatments for this difficult disease.

How do I find out about volunteering for drug trials?

Generally if you are attending a large MND clinic you will be kept informed about opportunities to participate. A good place to look for information about trials that are recruiting patients is the web pages of whichever national organization for MND is relevant to where you live (e.g. the MNDA in the UK, www.mndassociation.org.uk). A list is provided in Chapter 10, page 135. People often ask whether, if they live in Europe for example, they can travel to the USA to participate in clinical trials. While this is in theory possible, it is hardly ever practical. There are usually enough local patients who can be recruited, the frequent visits for assessment would essentially require emigration and it is unlikely that insurance companies would cover health care costs for someone with a disease such as MND who wishes to move to the USA.

What other kinds of MND research are being carried out apart from drug trials?

The same principles which apply to trials of new drug treatments can and should be applied to any management intervention in a disease. This is because we should know that resources are being used in the best way to benefit patients, that our treatments are not causing harm and because we wish to communicate to others, through publishing evidence, that there are things that can help. For example, as mentioned in Chapter 4, some patients with MND benefit from NIV. Because it is a relatively expensive treatment it has to be justified as a cost-effective and beneficial intervention. Evidence of benefit through a randomized trial of NIV has been published, allowing MND experts to argue the case that the investment of resources is justified.

One of the major areas for MND research at present is aimed at identifying tests which can improve early diagnosis and also aid in monitoring the disease progress. Such tests are known as **biomarkers**. It will be apparent from the discussion above that the successful execution of clinical trials in MND requires vast resources. If we had a biomarker, a simple non-invasive test of disease progression, it is hoped that drugs could be screened for their potential disease-modifying effect using small groups of patients. One area that is currently receiving a lot of attention is brain imaging. New methods of MRI scanning, described in Chapter 2, are being developed and tested in MND to see if we can detect changes in the brain pathways involved in motor function. Participating in research of new scanning techniques is one way of contributing to our understanding of MND. Most patients with MND will have experienced an MRI scan at the time of diagnosis. However, a research scan will differ in a number of ways. The environment will often be outside the normal hospital buildings and will probably seem more like a laboratory than a clinic. The scan itself will generally take longer, typically over 1 hour, because many different types of data are being collected. This means that patients with significant respiratory or bulbar involvement who have difficulty lying flat will not tolerate such scans and will not therefore be eligible. For any patient with MND, lying flat in a confined space may be uncomfortable and induce cramps. The researchers should have given careful thought to how to maintain the comfort of research subjects and will have sought approval for the research from the local ethics committee.

What are the rules governing DNA and tissue collection?

Much of what was learned about MND in the late nineteenth century and most of the twentieth century came from looking at the brain and spinal cord of patients who had died. This was and continues to be a vital way to understand what is going on in the nervous system in MND. In a previous era, when social relationships were more hierarchical, it was generally assumed that doctors always behaved for the best and there was very little requirement to justify post-mortem research or seek consent for the retention of human tissue after death. In the UK, a small number of highly publicized episodes in which it was revealed that the brains of patients, including many children, had been retained by pathology departments without the explicit consent of patients or their relatives led to widespread criticism of the medical profession for acting in a way that was perceived to be paternalistic and insensitive. This has led to much tighter regulation of the rules surrounding tissue collection and retention. The **Human Tissue Act (2004)** was enacted to update the law on organs and tissue to be more appropriate for twenty-first century society. It stipulates that tissue or organs cannot be taken or kept without consent other than for a Coroner to establish the cause of death. An overarching authority was set up to regulate post-mortems and research on human tissue, the **Human Tissue Authority**, http://www.hta.gov.uk/. The spirit of these reforms was intended to be positive and to improve public confidence so that people will be more willing to agree to valuable uses of tissue and organs such as research and transplantation.

Although it is a delicate subject, we have found that many patients ask us whether their brain and spinal cord would be useful to researchers. A few academic centres, specializing in neuropathological research, have established archives of brain material to aid research into MND (for a list in the UK see the MNDA website: http://www.mndassociation.org/research/dna_bank/ index.html). These brain archives or 'brain banks' are run by supervising committees who ensure that the material is collected ethically, stored appropriately and protected from misuse. Each committee will typically contain individuals dedicated to the protection of archival brain material because their research depends on it, as well as lay representatives and professional ethicists.

If a patient wishes to discuss the issue of brain donation we will make time in clinic to explain the process fully and also to obtain consent. The new law states that the wishes of the deceased individual should be honoured and therefore in theory family members cannot reverse a decision to donate once someone has died. In practice, however, it would be unusual for doctors to act in a way which would increase the suffering of bereaved relatives, and it is standard practice to obtain consent from the next of kin after death. Further information on donating human tissue can be obtained from the Human Tissue Authority and the MNDA.

DNA samples are frequently collected by doctors in MND clinics who wish to pursue research into the cause of MND. While many clinics have their own 'DNA collections', there is an increasing recognition that the power of genetic technology is best harnessed by groups of researchers working in cooperation. The UK research community has established a system for collecting DNA from individuals with MND and their relatives. Other collections have been established in the USA and elsewhere. The aim is to assemble several thousand samples with which to compare DNA samples from matched control individuals to look for patterns of gene variation which occur more frequently in MND patients and might give a clue as to the risk factors for the disease. People with MND who donate a blood sample for DNA extraction must be aware that the results of any genetic analyses will not be fed back to them directly by the researchers. Genetic studies in this context are aimed at solving the overall contribution of genes to the cause of MND. Any results of these endeavours will be published and allow individual doctors to test their own clinic patients where relevant.

In conclusion, in this chapter we have indicated some of the areas where people living with MND can participate in research and some of the advantages and difficulties associated with being a research subject. Whether the cause and cure of MND will be discovered in the near or remote future, it will only be achieved by a partnership between neurologists, neuroscientists and, very crucially, patients with MND.

8

Decision–making and remaining in control

Introduction

One of the most challenging aspects of living with MND is coping with a sense of loss of control. This arises from a combination of awareness that something serious is happening, that doctors do not know the cause, seem to have a limited ability to predict the course of the disease and offer no immediate prospect of a cure. This may produce a feeling akin to being on a ship without the ability to steer. Most patients feel that they wish to do something active and may feel frustrated by the lack of clear advice from health care professionals about how to 'fight' the disease. We have tried to emphasize in this book the importance of an active approach to nutrition, respiratory function and the management of disability. A crucial part of regaining some sense of control in the midst of a difficult situation is to plan for change by facing some key decisions head on. While this can naturally appear threatening at first, our experience is that most people find this process helpful because it allows an open discussion of the effects of MND on the individual, which can have the effect of reducing fear, both of the unknown and of aspects of the disease which are not relevant to an individual situation.

How can I make my wishes known?

We must make hundreds of choices each day. Most of these are simple matters such as what to wear and what to eat for lunch, and do not affect others. Making the wrong choice may be irritating, but it does not have lasting consequences. It can even be a valuable learning experience. However, things become more complex when our decisions affect other people or have a major impact on our future. For example, the decision to change jobs or stop working altogether will affect our family, our colleagues and our finances. The ability to make choices is central to remaining in control and taking charge of our lives. Choices about health and illness are among the most difficult we face as individuals and therefore the decisions we make are guided and supported by our doctor. Although, following discussion, this may lead to a joint decision being made about the best way to proceed, no treatment is ever given to an adult with mental capacity without full consent. The meaning of consent in this context is an understanding of the consequences of any decision. For a person living with MND there are many complex decisions to be made, and in each case support and guidance can be given by the care team. Even if communication has become more difficult, it is usually still possible for the wishes of the person with MND to be fully understood and respected.

Occasionally, unforeseen circumstances and medical emergencies may arise which require important decisions to be made in a situation where the person with MND is not able to communicate their wishes effectively. For example, other medical problems unrelated to MND such as a stroke or heart attack can impair communication or lead to unconsciousness. Occasionally people with MND may be admitted to hospital in an unstable or unconscious state due to a serious chest infection arising as a result of the disease itself. Even if such medical emergencies leave verbal or written communication intact, this will inevitably be a difficult time at which to process information, make decisions or communicate one's wishes in a calm and considered way. In such situations, doctors have an ethical and legal obligation to act in the best interests of the patient. The British Medical Association (BMA) states that it is good practice for relatives to be consulted when determining what is in the patients best interest. However, at present (see Mental Capacity Bill, below), relatives or next of kin do not have a legal right to make decisions on behalf of family members. What really helps both doctors and relatives in this situation is if the patient has given thought to what they would want to happen should they ever be in position where they cannot communicate their own wishes. The best way to do this is to record one's wishes in a written form called an Advance Directive (AD), also popularly referred to as a 'Living Will', or an 'advance decision to refuse treatment' in the Mental Capacity Act 2005 (see below).

What is an Advance Directive?

The following is only a brief explanation of the law; it is not a substitute for detailed legal advice or local policies. Individuals may wish to consult a solicitor or other legal advisor depending on their particular circumstances.

An AD is becoming widely accepted as a way for people to make their views known in relation to medical interventions. The courts have confirmed that if an individual states their wishes in advance these will be valid at the time treatment is being considered, even if that person is incapable of communicating.

Evidence from case law indicates that if the AD is ignored, this could result in a criminal charge of assault or a civil claim as it is in breach of the Human Rights Act (Article 8; the right to a private life). An AD only allows an individual to specify a *refusal* to some or all types of treatment, but not to be able to demand treatment where it would be medically inappropriate. Therefore, an AD *does not* enable an individual to make illegal requests such as euthanasia or assisted suicide. Neither does it enable a person to specify that, if unconscious, they do not want what is known as 'basic care' which includes warmth, shelter, pain relief, good hygiene, and food and nutrition offered by mouth. An AD cannot be used to request or demand specific types of treatment (*Burke v GMC*) or request anything with the primary purpose to hasten or bring about death. This is illegal and could result in criminal charges for medical personnel or carers.

Can anyone make an Advance Directive?

In order to be able to make an AD a person must:

- Be an adult, i.e. over the age of 18

- Be able to understand the consequences of their decisions

- Have the mental capacity to refuse treatment. By law it is assumed that every one over the age of 18 has capacity unless there is evidence to the contrary

- Make the AD without pressure or persuasion from anyone else.

An AD may only be changed or updated by the individual to whom the AD specifically refers.

How does an Advance Directive differ from an Advance Statement?

An Advance Statement enables a person to state their general views and preferences about different forms of treatment and can be used to record 'personal philosophies' or religious beliefs. It can enable carers to understand the values and priorities of the person they are caring for. An Advance Statement could be used to guide and inform health care professionals when considering treatment decisions. It may also be used to nominate someone to act as an advocate if the need arises. Unlike an AD, an Advance Statement would not legally bind medical personnel to a particular treatment or course of action if they felt that it was not in the best interests of the patient. An Advance Statement may only give guidance; it is not a legally binding document.

Does an Advanced Directive have to be signed by a witness?

It is essential to have a written, signed and dated document. If the owner of the AD is unable to write or hold a pen, then a thumb print could be used. It is also advisable that an AD is reviewed and updated regularly to ensure that there is no doubt that it represents the current views of the person with MND and that they have not changed their mind since it was initially written. Changes in medical technology which may not have been considered when the AD was first written have the potential to influence individual choice. It is difficult to specify how often an AD should be reviewed. This will depend on individual circumstances, and could vary from 3 to 12 months, at which time it should be re-signed and dated to indicate that there has been no change. In law, for an AD to state a refusal of life-sustaining treatment it must be (1) in writing, and (2) signed in the presence of a witness, who must also sign the document. In addition, asking your doctor to sign it is a good idea as it verifies that a well informed professional judges that you have capacity to make an AD and that a full discussion of the implications has taken place. Your doctor may also wish to have a copy for the medical notes. It is not necessary to pay a solicitor to draw up and witness an AD, but there may be individual circumstances where this becomes necessary, such as when there is a dispute about mental capacity.

What if I wish to change my mind?

It is the absolute right of anyone making an AD that they may change their mind about its contents at any time. If changes are made, it is important to keep track of who holds a copy as the 'out of date' AD must be retrieved before issuing new instructions to avoid confusion. Any new instructions must be signed and dated. The Mental Capacity Act 2005 (see below) states that an AD can be withdrawn at any time and that this does not have to be in writing.

How do you make an Advance Directive?

An AD must be made in writing. A casual remark made in passing does not constitute the basis for an AD. If verbal instructions are given and are witnessed, these should be respected and upheld in the normal course of events. However, it is possible that any instructions only given verbally may be ignored in an emergency situation, as refusal to treat may be in conflict with a health care professional's duty of care. Consider the following hypothetical example. Fred stops breathing at home while gardening and a neighbour calls an ambulance. When the crew assesses Fred and decide to initiate resuscitation they may ignore his wife who says: 'Stop! Fred said he did not want this to happen, he just wants to be left alone'. It is impossible for the paramedic crew to make a quick decision based purely on a comment from one person, and without knowing Fred's history or personal beliefs or the relationship between Fred and his wife! They simply have a 'duty of care' to every patient to do what is best in a particular situation. Hence, their choice to resuscitate, unless there is a set of written instructions to guide them in another direction.

There is no required legal wording for completing an AD. However, it is important that it is clear and succinct. Very wordy documents may be ambiguous and open to misinterpretation at a time when clarity and accuracy are crucial. An AD does not necessarily have to be drawn up by someone with a legal qualification. Although solicitors are willing to assist people in this regard, our experience is that the resulting document is sometimes vague and 'off-the-peg', and does not address the specific needs of people with MND. It is actually very easy for people to make their own AD, and a number of websites provide templates. Some of these are listed in Chapter 10. However, the assistance of an MND specialist clinic team is advisable as they will have the necessary experience to guide patients through the different decision points in their journey with MND.

The principal aim of making an AD for people living with MND is to remain in control of their care, particularly in the late stages of the disease. In law, an AD is not actually valid if the person to whom it refers retains the capacity to make decisions. ADs are therefore only used when the person living with MND is both critically ill and unable to communicate in any way. This is actually a relatively rare situation, but incorrect decisions at this time can have devastating consequences. It is normal to find the process of discussing and making an AD very challenging. In the early stages of an illness such as MND it is difficult to confront issues that seem more relevant to terminal care. An AD is there to provide insurance against events that are very unlikely to occur in practice, and most people find it difficult to relate these to the context of their own journey with MND. In this respect, an AD is like any other insurance policy which we hope we will never have to call upon.

To meet the needs of people living with MND, an AD should include some statement about a number of situations, some of which are generally applicable to all terminal illness, some of which are more specific to MND. One of the main aims underlying the points discussed below is to establish the circumstances under which people with MND wish to be admitted to hospital. This is a very individual matter. Given that MND is a terminal illness, many people express a strong desire to have all of their treatment at home and, in practice, very few people (perhaps 1–2 per cent from our clinic) die in hospital. We also generally prefer patients with significant disability from MND to avoid inpatient hospital admissions as this also increases the chance of contracting a chest infection. However, many people are willing to consider hospital or hospice admission at different stages of the illness, and this choice should be clearly recorded.

The AD should consist of a series of clearly worded statements about situations which may arise in the course of MND.

◆ An AD should contain some simple information making it clear who 'owns' it, i.e. who is the person to whom it refers, and also who is the principal contact in times of emergency (which may be the same as the next of kin).

◆ One of the most common situations to consider is what to do in the event of a chest infection developing. Most people feel comfortable taking antibiotics by mouth with a prescription from their family doctor to deal with a simple chest infection. However, if the infection is not controlled by oral antibiotics, a decision will have to be taken as to whether the treatment should continue in hospital with intravenous therapy or not. This is both a very individual decision and one that might change depending on the degree of disease progression. Some patients with mild to moderate disability will have no reservations about hospital treatment. Many people at the end of their lives wish to remain at home, and admission to an acute hospital for intravenous therapy for what may potentially be a terminal event therefore goes against their wishes. An AD will therefore need to be revised from time to time.

◆ In a situation where someone is at the end of life but unconscious, there is sometimes anxiety about whether a patient who cannot drink will experience discomfort from dehydration. This sometimes precipitates hospital admission because the facilities do not exist in the community for giving fluids intravenously. Obviously if a PEG is in place this does not arise. In general, in MND, discomfort from dehydration is not an issue and should not be the prime reason for hospital admission. A hospice is likely to be a more comfortable and appropriate environment. However, given that it may be possible to have intravenous fluids at home, it is good practice to record a preference if there is a strong feeling about this issue.

◆ Morphine and its related drugs are commonly used for symptom control in terminal care. Morphine can have wide-ranging beneficial effects including treating pain, promoting comfort, reducing anxiety, relieving breathlessness and enhancing sleep. However, a significant side effect of morphine and related drugs is to depress both the rate and depth of breathing. In patients with MND, in whom respiratory function may already be impaired, this can lead to deterioration. Given that these drugs are only likely to be used to address symptoms very late in an illness, there will not usually be a conflict between the good effects of morphine and the bad effects. However, it is important for medical staff to know that they are acting according to wishes of the patient and that possible negative effects of morphine are accepted by all concerned as a justified price to pay for good symptom relief.

◆ Good care at the end of life can be achieved in a number of different settings including one's own home, a hospice or hospital. Most people have a strong view about where they wish to be cared for. For many people this is their own home, but some people, for example those who do not have close family or friends nearby, feel more secure knowing that they will be cared for in a hospice or hospital if necessary. Whatever the reason, it is important to include a clear statement about preferences for place of care in the AD. If there is an absolute view that there are no circumstances in which a person wishes to go to hospital, this should be made clear.

◆ Perhaps the most difficult situation for people to consider relates to what might happen in a situation where there is complete cessation of breathing and heart function. While this might happen for reasons unrelated to MND such as a heart attack, mostly this is a terminal event caused by MND itself. It should be stressed that for most people this is not a sudden event like a 'cardiac arrest' but a gradual process of slipping away into a coma, which is generally peaceful. However, in the unusual circumstance in which there appears to be a sudden unexpected cessation of breathing at a time and in a place that were not anticipated, there may be an attempt by paramedics or trained bystanders to initiate cardiopulmonary resuscitation as would be natural in an emergency situation. However, people with MND who are resuscitated from a cardiorespiratory arrest are very unlikely to be able to breathe independently again and face the prospect of a more prolonged terminal phase of their illness during which they are permanently attached to a respirator via a tracheostomy. For most of our patients this represents a situation that they wish to avoid and does not equate to a dignified and peaceful end to their life. Therefore, even though it is a rare event which usually occurs in an emergency situation where there is panic and uncertainty about what to do, the consequences can be very devastating. A clear statement in an AD indicating that someone wishes to have all care to support their well-being and comfort but not to have their life artificially prolonged by invasive (i.e. tracheostomy-assisted) ventilation is an important way of avoiding this outcome.

Once an AD has been made, and signed and dated by the person to whom it refers and also by a witness, it is important to be clear about how many copies have been made and their location. In the event that the AD is changed or rewritten, the first version should be destroyed. We generally advise the following:

- Keep one copy at home. The Lions Club, www.lions.org.uk/miab.htm, can provide a 'message in a bottle'. The AD is placed in the bottle which is then kept in the refrigerator. A sticker with a green cross placed on the front and back doors alerts any emergency services that there is important medical information in the fridge, chosen because it is normally in the kitchen and easy to locate. Some GP practices routinely use the message in a bottle scheme, but these can also be obtained directly from the Lions Club. Some people decide to keep one copy on their person or in a hand bag.

- Give one copy to your next of kin.

- Give one copy to your GP for your medical notes.

- In some areas the local ambulance control will be happy to indicate on their database the fact that someone has an AD. Thus if an ambulance is ever called they will be alerted to the fact that someone in the household has an AD.

In the UK, a copy of an AD can also be sent to NHS Direct which now has a national database and a system for flagging up special instructions such as an AD.

The Mental Capacity Act 2005

Providing the AD complies with all the above recommendations, doctors are duty bound to respect it. From April 2007, the Mental Capacity Act 2005 has been implemented and forms the legal framework. In the Act, ADs are referred to as 'Advance Decisions to Refuse Treatment'.

The Act is underpinned by five key principles:

- Everyone is presumed to be capable of making decisions about their lives unless it is proved otherwise.

- Individuals must be given support to enable them to make their own decisions before it is concluded that they are unable to do so.

- Individual decisions must be respected even if these may seem to be eccentric.

- All decisions made on behalf of a person (without capacity to make their own decisions) must be in their best interests.

- Any intervention on behalf of a person without capacity should be the least restrictive to their basic rights and freedom.

Each of the above sections of the Act is covered in great depth. The area of most interest in relation to ADs is where the Act enables an individual to designate a decision maker, called a 'Lasting Power of Attorney' (LPA), who can act on behalf of someone if they lose capacity to make their own decisions. This is similar to the current 'Enduring Power of Attorney' (EPA); however, in addition, the new Act enables the LPA to make decisions about health and welfare. This includes an advance refusal of treatment. For further information, see 'Mental Capacity Act 2005', published by The Stationary Office Limited, or read the Act directly at http://www.opsi.gov.uk/acts/acts2005/20050009.htm.

Conclusions

In this chapter we have emphasized that in a disease such as MND where there are constant changes to adapt to, meeting decisions head on can help maintain a sense of control. Important decisions relate to many points in the journey with MND, not just at the end of life. The law has recently clarified the validity of advance decisions to refuse life-sustaining treatment. We encourage people living with MND to see ADs as an insurance policy, like any other, to protect against an unwanted but rare event.

9

Caring for people living with motor neuron disease

Introduction

Caring for someone with MND is a challenge whether you are a health care professional or a close family member or friend. Anyone who made the marriage vow 'in sickness and in health', however sincerely meant, would never have been able to envisage that a disease such as MND would transform their world. Occasionally caring for a person with MND can be too challenging; relationships suffer, the health of the carer deteriorates and the whole situation occasionally breaks down. However, for the most part, people placed in the position of caring for a loved one manage to come through with enormous bravery and resilience in which the journey through the illness is, perhaps, the most difficult, but one of many challenges that people face in their relationships.

MND has an enormous impact on family, friends and colleagues, and could never be described as a disease that affects an individual in isolation. As with the disease itself, which develops insidiously, the process of caring for someone with MND can have subtle beginnings. At first it may just be providing a steadying hand going up a step. The impact of bad news at the time of diagnosis may be just as significant for a partner or spouse as it is for the person with MND, and it should be a shared burden. The realization that life will not be the same again may feel like crossing a bridge into a land from which there is no return. As the disease progresses, what is mainly emotional support may grow into full 24-hour care, a full-time job that was never anticipated. People may not feel qualified to take on such a role, which is understandable when one considers that formal experience or qualifications would be required for a full-time carer on the open job market. This chapter aims to explore the experience and anxieties associated with caring for someone with MND and encourage partners, carers and friends to seek support and information for themselves.

Patient's perspective

Alan was referred to our clinic by the local hospice team. He had developed MND in his early 40s and had slowly progressed over a period of 10 years to a state in which he was dependent on help for all activities of daily living. For a number of years he had lived with his girlfriend, Joanna, who was his full-time carer. She looked after his daily needs in an extraordinarily dedicated way. For some years she had not had a holiday, and arrangements were made for Alan to be admitted to the local hospice for a week of respite care while Joanna had a break. In order to make sure that the hospice understood Alan's needs, Joanna helpfully wrote a 50-page guide, carefully documenting his likes and dislikes and making sure there were instructions to cover every minute of the day.

Joanna did not find it easy to relax on holiday and, worse, when she returned, she did not like what she found. Many of her precise instructions had not been followed by the hospice. Joanna was sure that Alan was in a worse condition than when she had left him and had contracted a chest infection in the hospice. She vowed never to give up his care to someone else again.

Caring for someone with severe disability can be an all-consuming thing especially if it is as part of a loving partnership. Carers can sometimes feel that they are the only people who can provide what is needed. Although this is understandable, the state of co-dependence that can arise can have damaging effects. The reality is that a change of environment can be disruptive, especially to someone who is unwell. It is important to have realistic expectations of what is available and not to seek perfection from a system that has to cater for all and can never replicate the one-to-one care available at home.

What is a 'carer'?

The term 'carer' is used in many ways, but the recognized definition is someone who is caring for a partner, friend or child but does not have a paid contract of work. This care normally takes place in the home of the person being cared for. Interestingly, the 2001 Census identified that there were 5.2 million carers living in England and Wales. That equates to 1 in 10 of the population. One million of these carers provide more than 50 hours of care per week. These statistics reveal much about the structure of our society and the impact of severe illness on people's lives. Therefore, carers rather than the NHS and Social Services provide the vast majority of care for people in this country, and their contribution is vastly undervalued. It is not surprising that studies have shown that being a carer is associated with higher than average rates of both physical and mental ill health. If carers do not seek help and support, there is a risk that their social horizons contract and they may become socially isolated.

Patient's perspective

Don and Angela had been married for 35 years when Don was diagnosed with MND at the age of 63. Their life was very well ordered and predictable. Don, a chartered accountant, was exceptionally hard working and thrived on 16-hour days. He had converted the upper floor of their semi-detached house into a home office. They had no children and their circle of friends consisted of members of the local golf club and church. Generally they were a very well respected couple, but it was recognized that they valued their privacy and generally led a quiet life. They had been unable to have children and Angela had devoted herself over the years to keeping the house spotlessly clean and well ordered.

When Don was diagnosed with MND, he and Angela reacted in different ways. Don, never a man who found it easy to express his emotions, retreated more into his work. Angela, one of life's organizers, began to plan for adaptations to the home. The house was suddenly full of OTs, builders, MNDA visitors and all sorts of other well-meaning people. Don became irritated with all the fuss and Angela rapidly became frustrated with the apparently slow pace at which things were being done. However, they did not seem to be talking about the things that really mattered. After the first few months it became clear that Don's illness was progressing quite rapidly and he was no longer able to travel to work. For the first time in 35 years Don and Angela were spending every day together and Don, a proud and self-sufficient man, needed help for everyday things. He found it very upsetting that his wife had to help him with the lavatory in particular. We had many conversations with them in clinic in which they voiced their frustrations with each other and with MND. Their world had truly been turned upside down, and a very stable and well ordered pattern of life had been turned into one characterized by invasion of privacy and a major reorientation in the dynamics of their relationship. Although this was clearly a strain for them both, soon after Don died Angela told us that because of MND 'I really got to know him for the first time'.

What rights do carers have?

In 2000 the Carers and Disabled Children Act allowed carers who were aged 16 or over, and provided a regular and substantial amount of care for someone aged 18 or over, to have the right to an assessment of their needs carried out by Social Services. If there is more than one carer providing regular care in a household, both carers are entitled to an assessment. In 2004 the Carers Equal Opportunities Act set out to increase the rights of carers. If a carer wishes to undertake study or leisure activity, this should be taken into account as part of the assessment. The aim of this is to encourage carers to have time to pursue their own interests. The health and well-being of a carer is of paramount importance and if the carer becomes overtired, stressed or injured they will be unable to care, and the whole situation can reach crisis point.

Sandra developed MND when she was 41, and the disease progressed quite rapidly. She had a background of depression, and the whole thing was such a dreadful shock that she retreated into a shell and was difficult to reach. After the first few visits she no longer wished to come to clinic and remained at home and took to her bed. Sandra was married to Dave who worked as a manager of a video shop. He also found the diagnosis very traumatic and, though he seemed to be finding it difficult to cope, refused our offer of counselling. After some months, we were contacted by Sandra's 16-year-old daughter Rachel. We learned that Dave had started drinking heavily and staying out late. He absolutely forbade any discussion of Sandra's illness and refused to acknowledge the fact that she was dying. Sandra's 13-year-old son Steven was having a difficult time at school but at home mostly stayed in his room playing computer games in the evening. The third child, Siobhan, was just 6 years old when Sandra was diagnosed. She would bounce into her mother's bedroom and ask why her mother was not getting up. No answers were forthcoming and Siobhan began to show signs of anxiety at school. Rachel became the main carer for Sandra until she died 15 months after her disease started. This coincided with a time when Rachel was taking her GCSE exams and in many ways being a surrogate mother for her little sister.

One of the most neglected groups of carers in society are children looking after their parents. Although the story of Sarah and her family demonstrates that within the family structure there are incredible resources and very positive forms of behaviour in action, the level of responsibility taken on by Rachel raises concerns about the effect on her.

How to avoid a crisis point?

Caring is, almost by definition, a selfless act, so people tend to place the needs of those they are caring for above their own. While this is completely understandable, carers must always ask themselves whether what they are doing **now** is sustainable for weeks, months or years to come. It is not a sign of weakness or failure to accept help and support, more a sign of good planning and self-preservation which, in the long term, will benefit both the carer and the person being cared for. The type and amount of help accepted is entirely up to the individual and naturally depends on local availability of resources. The following are examples of different types of care that may be available.

- **Residential respite care** where the person being cared for goes to stay in suitable accommodation for a fixed period of time. It may be in the local community hospital, disability centre, hospice or even a hotel.

- **Domiciliary care** occurs at home. Depending on individual agreements, this may mean paid care staff from an agency assisting with the daily needs of the person living with MND, either at set times during the day or for a block of time which should reflect the carer's needs as well as those of the person with MND.

- **Day care** enables individuals to be cared for out of the home environment, returning home in the afternoon. The frequency of this will vary according to individual needs, but is typically once or twice a week. Day care often provides ongoing assessment for the person attending, as well as respite for their carer, providing some much needed free time. In an ideal world, the carer would be able to go and pamper themselves with a new 'hair do' or a massage. Sadly, in reality, this time is most often spent dashing about doing all the chores you do not normally have time for.

Accepting any of the above can be very difficult for a number of reasons. Many carers tell us that they feel a tremendous amount of **guilt**. They know that they may not have much time left with their partner or friend and therefore any time spent apart seems wrong. For the carers to go out and 'enjoy' themselves does not bring them the same pleasure it once did. Some carers tell us that they are really 'torn' because the person they are caring for has become dependent on them. They are told that no-one else can care for them in the same way and no-one else knows what to do. In one respect this is true; over a period of time two people become attuned to one another. They have worked out how to do things together by problem solving, often resulting in excellent team work. No matter how true this is, the team may break down due to exhaustion or stress if preventative measures are not put into place. By slowly introducing 'outside helpers' and enabling them to get to know the person living with MND, the circle of trust may gradually grow to incorporate other people as well as the main carer. Being able to share some of the burden of care may make the situation more sustainable in the long term and prevent a crisis.

 Patient's perspective

Carol was a 55-year-old teacher with a love of antiques. When she was referred to the MND clinic with a confirmed diagnosis she was only suffering from foot drop and it was unclear how her disease would progress. She came alone for the first visit, commenting that she had rowed with her husband that morning and he had decided to stay at home.

We got to know Carol well over the next 5 years as it became clear that the rate of progression of her MND was much slower than average, but she always came to clinic alone. She was able to continue working and, despite significant stiffness in her legs, did not lose the ability to walk. One day we received a letter from her husband Martin. It was very angry in tone and accused us of not being clear about Carol's prognosis. He admitted that at the time the diagnosis was made their marriage was in great trouble and he had been about to leave Carol for someone else. When he heard that she had a 'terminal illness' he decided that, despite their troubles, he would stand by her and help her through to the end. Five years later she was still relatively well and he had lost the chance of happiness with someone else. The natural feeling of guilt that Martin experienced because he was having an extra-marital affair had been compounded when Carol was diagnosed with MND and this had prevented him from following his own path in life.

We were never able to understand Martin's needs as a carer because we had never met him. His information about MND came from the Internet and his GP, and unfortunately did not match the clinical pattern of Carol's illness. Whatever the difficulties of a relationship that is breaking down, leaving someone who is ill may be so socially unacceptable that it may literally be impossible.

Interestingly, we have encountered a number of examples of estranged and even divorced couples who, when one partner develops MND, come back together again so that the person with MND can be cared for. The bond between people who cannot manage to live together under normal circumstances can be resurrected in adversity.

Where can you seek support?

Each carer has their own needs and so will seek individual support solutions. Just knowing what kind of support is available in your area may well be enough of a reassurance that help is there if needed.

◆ **The Motor Neuron Disease Association** (MNDA) is the best place to start. The excellent MNDA website, www.mndassociation.org, offers a great deal of information and there is also a Help Line number, 08457 626262. The MNDA has a vast network of support across the country. Most areas have a local branch of the MNDA which can give individual support to both the person living with MND and their partner, family and friends. The MNDA also fund **MND Care Centres, Regional Care**

Advisors, Association Visitors and **MND Local branches,** all of which are there to offer ongoing advice and support to people living with MND.

- **Health and Social Care.** Your local office can organize an initial visit and carry out a Carers Assessment. The Care Manager will be able to discuss the support that they can provide.

- **Carers UK** www.carersuk.org has the power to lobby on behalf of carers and also has a forum for carers to communicate on-line. This is a good way to share experiences and receive advice and support from people in similar situations.

- **The Carers Centre** www.thecarerscentre.org is a national network which gives carers support and information including practical assistance in filling out forms and applying for grants.

What happens when caring comes to an end?

Bereavement is a long-term process. It will be clear that caring for MND can take up a significant amount of time, and the pattern of life can become reoriented so that many normal activities are put 'on hold'. Re-establishing a regular pattern of work and leisure brings its own challenges. There are a variety of useful sources of information for the bereaved including http:// www.crusebereavementcare.org.uk/. It is remarkable how many people who are touched by the experience of caring for someone with MND ultimately become MNDA volunteers and retain a significant contact with the disease and its impact.

If there is just one simple message from this chapter it is that being a responsible carer means looking after yourself as well as someone else. If your health or psychological well-being is threatened, this has major implications for the person for whom you care.

10

Useful information

Much of the information in this section is most easily accessed via the Internet. For those without access to a computer we have included telephone contact details.

How do I stay informed?

Internet-based sources of information

There are many sources of information about MND and related disorders on the Internet. We have only included below those sites with which we are familiar and for which the web address is likely to remain constant over time. The Internet is a great force for freedom of information, but it is important to remember that not all information contained on websites is from a reliable source. For those who are new to the Internet, we suggest you start with the respected sources of information listed below.

Motor Neuron Disease Association (UK): http://www.mndassociation.org

* Provides a wide range of general information about MND. Information specific to the UK, such as the location of MNDA-funded Care Centres is also included.

* MNDA Help Line 08457 626262.

ALS Association (USA): http://www.alsa.org/

* This is a very comprehensive site which has up to date information about research as well as factual information about the disease itself.

Synapse (USA): http://www.synapsepls.org/

* A website specifically devoted to primary lateral sclerosis.

The International Alliance of ALS/MND Associations:
http://www.alsmndalliance.org/

◆   This provides international information which can link anyone living with
    MND to the clinics and organizations relevant to their locality.

DIPex (UK): http://www.alsmndalliance.org/index.shtml

◆   **DIPEx** is a site devoted to personal experiences of health and illness.
    You can watch, listen to or read interviews with people suffering from
    various diseases including MND and find reliable information on treat-
    ment choices and where to find support.

If I just needed to know one number what would it be?

For most queries and advice we would recommend calling the MNDA Help
Line 08457 626262. The operators are highly trained to give advice and they
have a great resource of up to date information. The help line operators are
totally in tune with people living with MND. They are therefore able to give
sound, appropriate advice.

How do I find my nearest specialist MND clinic?

In the UK, the MNDA website has a list of specialist clinics. In the USA, the
ALSA holds a similar list. Elsewhere in the world, the International Alliance of
MND Associations maintains a list.

How do I continue driving?
What is a blue badge?

http://www.direct.gov.uk/en/DisabledPeople/MotoringAndTransport/

The scheme operates throughout the UK and within the EU. It provides a
range of parking benefits for people with a disability who have walking difficulties. The badge-holder may be either the driver or the passenger.

Where can I park?

You can download a map of all the blue badge parking areas from the above
link to the UK Government website. The badge may only be used for on-street
parking. It includes free use of parking meters and pay-and-display bays.
Badge-holders may also be exempt from limits on parking times imposed on

others and can park for up to 3 hours on yellow lines (except where there is a ban on loading or unloading or other restrictions).

Do I qualify?

Most people living with MND will qualify for a blue badge. Some people are reluctant to apply at first, but find it really useful once they do!

Where can I obtain a blue badge?

Each County Council will work slightly differently, but a good place to start is to call your local Town Hall which will be able to give you the correct contact number. The County Council works within the Department of Transport guidelines, and the Disabled Parking department will send you an application form. Verification of your diagnosis will be requested from your GP before a Blue Badge is issued. The whole process is likely to take approximately 3 weeks.

Can I still drive?

Having the diagnosis of MND does not automatically stop you from driving. However, you must inform the DVLA and your insurance company. Failure to notify the DVLA of a medical condition or disability that affects your driving is a criminal offence and is punishable by a fine of up to £1000. If a medical practitioner advises you not to drive, you must surrender your licence. However, you can do this voluntarily at any point.

For telephone advice call: 0870 600 0301

The DVLA have a comprehensive website for more information: www.dvla. org.uk, and can be contacted at:

Drivers Medical Group
DVLA
Swansea
SA99 1TU

Can I travel abroad?

Most patients with MND can travel abroad if they have good respiratory function. Common sense dictates that the decision to fly is best made after consultation with your neurologist. Some patients who have reduced respiratory function, including those using NIV, will be able to fly, but should discuss this with their doctors. It is worth considering the following factors that might represent a threat to a person with MND who flies in an aircraft:

- Most commercial aircraft travel at 30 000–35 000 ft. Although the cabin is pressurized, it is still equivalent to being at about 7000 ft. This slightly reduces the amount of oxygen which gets into the lungs. For a fit healthy person with no lung disease this is not significant, but for anyone who has poor respiratory function this small change can make a big difference. Patients with MND who have no respiratory symptoms (i.e. can lie flat, sleep well and are not short of breath) will generally encounter no problems.

- Aircraft are notorious harbingers of viruses and other infections, and there is a slightly increased risk of developing a respiratory tract infection for any passenger. This should be taken into account when deciding whether to fly.

- The risk of developing a clot in the veins of the leg (deep vein thrombosis or DVT) arises through a combination of restricted space to move about and a slight concentration of the blood due to the low pressure in the cabin. The added restriction to mobility experienced by people with MND increases this risk further. Compression socks improve the return of blood to the heart and lower the risk of DVT. We advise people with MND to avoid alcohol when flying as this increases the risk of dehydration. One tablet of aspirin taken the day before flying can reduce this risk considerably and, unless there is a specific medical reason why aspirin cannot be taken (allergy, stomach ulcers or interaction with other drugs), it should be considered by all patients with MND who fly. This should be discussed with your doctor.

- Flying is an exhausting business for anyone. Airlines are only too happy to facilitate the passage of customers with disability and should be made aware of specific needs at the time of booking. Even if a wheelchair is not necessary for everyday use, it can be invaluable when negotiating airport terminal buildings. Airlines will arrange for a wheelchair and a porter to be available.

Once on the ground, living with MND should be no different from home, although facilities for people with disability will vary enormously, even in the 'developed' world. Some simple fact finding before travel will pay dividends. http://www.dialuk.info and http://www.radar.org.uk are good places to find out about travel for people with disabilities.

The website http://www.doctorbabel.com/ offers a service where you can enter your medical details which can be translated into a document in most of the common languages. This can be printed off for you to take on your travels.

Obtaining travel insurance should not be a problem for people with MND but may require some research. It is essential to be adequately covered and to keep you insurance company informed of your medical history. The MNDA website contains up to date information about companies which are happy to insure people with MND. In the EU, emergency health cover is obtained with a European Health Insurance Card (EHIC) which entitles you to reduced cost, sometimes free, medical treatment.

Accessing benefits

How do I find out about the benefits I am entitled to?

Benefits can be a total mystery. It is important to get sound advice. Initially call the benefits enquiry line, 0800 882200, who will explain your entitlement to benefits and then send out the appropriate forms.

How do I fill out the forms?

Once the forms have been sent to you, they can look daunting. Indeed, your claim may be influenced by the way you fill out the form. So it is best to seek advice and assistance. Many people have found the Citizens Advice Bureau (CAB) helpful. CABs provide free, independent and confidential advice on a range of legal and monetary issues. They will provide guidance through the application forms. Each area will have a local CAB. The national office is 0207 833 2181. No advice is given out on this number, but they will be able to give you details of your local office.

Citizens Advice
Myddelton House
115–123 Pentonville Road
London
N1 9LZ
http://www.citizensadvice.org.uk

Am I eligible for a grant to adapt my home?

There is a grant known as the Disabled Facilities Grant (DFG). People with a permanent or substantial disability may be eligible. The grant comes from your local or city council.

Applicants are subject to a financial assessment.

Who carries out the assessment?

Your community OTs from the Health and Social Care Team will visit you and carry out an assessment of your needs. They will be able to advise on whether the work you are proposing to carry out is both necessary and appropriate to meet your needs.

Where can I get support as a carer? (see Chapter 9)

http://www.carers.org

http://www.thecarescentre.org

Practical advice for people with disabilities

DIAL UK is a national advice line with 130 local branches. This enables them to provide local disability information, advice and support.

It offers a range of cost-effective services including:

◆ a disability information database and monthly information service

◆ support for welfare rights advisers

◆ management support

◆ training.

Dial UK

Telephone 01302 310 123

Fax 01302 310404

Text phone 01302 310 123

http://www.dialuk.info

DIAL UK

St Catherine's
Tickhill Road
Doncaster
South Yorkshire
DN4 8QN

RADAR is a national network of disability organizations and disabled people which was established to campaign on disability rights issues. The website http://www.radar.org.uk has a lot of useful information about benefits and accessing help.

RADAR
12 City Forum
250 City Road
London
EC1V 8AF

By phone: 020 7250 3222

By fax: 020 7250 0212

By minicom: 020 7250 4119

By e-mail: radar@radar.org.uk

Index